DEADLY DAFFODILS
TOXIC CATERPILLARS

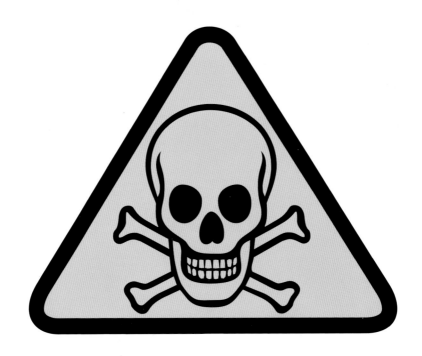

DEADLY DAFFODILS
TOXIC CATERPILLARS

The Family Guide to Preventing and
Treating Accidental Poisoning Inside and
Outside the Home

CHRISTOPHER P. HOLSTEGE, M.D. and **CAROL ANN TURKINGTON**

STEWART, TABORI & CHANG ▲ NEW YORK

Published in 2006 by Stewart, Tabori & Chang
An imprint of Harry N. Abrams, Inc.

Library of Congress Cataloging-in-Publication Data:
Holstege, Christopher P.
  Deadly daffodils, toxic caterpillars : a family safety guide to preventing and treating accidental poisoning inside and outside the home / Christopher P. Holstege and Carol Ann Turkington.
       p. cm.
  Includes index.
  ISBN-13: 978-1-58479-492-9
  ISBN-10: 1-58479-492-5
  1. Poisons--Safety measures--Popular works. 2. Poisons--Treatment--Popular works.
I. Turkington, Carol. II. Title.

RA1213.H65 2006
615.9'02--dc22

                                                                        2006009686

Notice: This book is intended as a reference guide, not a medical guide to self-treat-ment. If you suspect you have a medical condition or medical emergency, you should contact a health-care practitioner right away. If you are under treatment for any med-ical condition, do not change your treatment program without consulting with and get-ting the consent of your doctor.

Editor: Debora Yost
Designer: Galen Smith and Jessi Rymill
Production Manager: Jane Searle

Photograph credits: Page 98: © Jan De Laet, www.plantsystematics.com. Pages 103–10: © John Plischke. Page 119 (top): © William Flaxington. Page 119 (middle): © Jason Penny. Page 121: © David Cooper.

The text of this book was composed in Trade Gothic.

Printed and bound in China
10 9 8 7 6 5 4 3 2 1

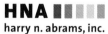
HNA
harry n. abrams, inc.
a subsidiary of La Martinière Groupe
115 West 18th Street
New York, NY 10011
www.hnabooks.com

CONTENTS

Find-It-Fast Directory   8
of Common Poisoning Hazards

Introduction   17
A Book for Every Household

1 **Poisoning Basics**   21
First Aid and Prevention

2 **Avoid Accidental Overdose**   33
Medications and Herbs

3 **Let Them Be**   63
Toxic Plants, Shrubs, Trees, and Mushrooms

4 **Steer Clear**   113
Poisonous Snakes and Toads

5 **Don't Get Stung**   125
Dangerous Insects

6 **Danger—Don't Touch!**   155
Chemicals

7 **Be Careful In There**   185
Toxic Water Creatures

8 **Eat, Drink, and Be Wary**   197
Food Poisoning

9 **Keep Baby Safe**   249
Poisons in the Nursery and Playroom

10 **Protect Your Pets**   265
Safeguards for the Curious

11 **Resources**   288

Index   304

FIND-IT-FAST DIRECTORY
OF COMMON POISONING HAZARDS

A

37 Acetaminophen
157 Alcohol
268 Alcohol (and pets)
176 Aluminum phosphide
214 Anisakiasis
39 Antianxiety drugs
40 Anticonvulsant drugs
41 Antidepressants
158 Antifreeze
268 Antifreeze (and pets)
43 Anti-inflammatory drugs
251 Art supplies
44 Aspirin
159 Automatic dishwasher soap
66 Azalea

B

215 Bacillus cereus
162 Batteries
126 Bee sting
67 Belladonna
168 Benzene
45 Birth control pills
161 Bleach
215 Botulism
122 Bufo toad

C

218   Campylobacteriosis

175   Carbamates

162   Carbon monoxide

133   Caterpillar stings

186   Catfish sting

166   Caustics

59   Chaparral

67   Chinaberry tree

270   Chocolate (and pets)

68   Christmas rose

220   Ciguatera

70   Clematis

45   Clonidine

55   Codeine

46   Cold medications

59   Comfrey

120   Copperhead bite

120   Coral snake bite

114   Cottonmouth bite

71   Crocus, autumn

222   Cryptosporidiosis

224   Cyclosporiasis

D

72   Daffodil

72   Death camas

177 **Diquat**

166 **Drain cleaner**

73 **Dumbcane**

168 **Duplicating fluid**

E

225 **E. coli**

59 **Ephedra**

59 **Eucalyptus oil**

F

55 **Fentanyl**

273 **Fertilizers (and pets)**

273 **Flea repellent (and pets)**

197 **Food poisoning**

168 **Formaldehyde**

74 **Foxglove**

168 **Furniture polish**

G

281 **Garlic (and pets)**

168 **Gasoline**

60 **Germander**

228 **Giardiasis**

283 **Grapes (and pets)**

H

48 **Heart medications**

76 **Hemlock**

231 Hepatitis A

56 Herbal products

282 Herbicides (and pets)

77 Holly

276 Houseplants (and pets)

78 Hyacinth

168 Hydrocarbons

55 Hydrocodone

I

43 Ibuprofen

125 Insect sting

50 Iron

52 Isoniazid

79 Ivy

J

80 Jack-in-the-pulpit

187 Jellyfish sting

81 Jerusalem cherry

82 Jessamine

83 Jimsonweed

84 Jonquil

K

60 Kava

170 Kerosene

132 Killer bees

L

168   Lamp oil

253   Lead

279   Lighter fluid (and pets)

84   Lily of the valley

233   Listeriosis

140   Lyme disease

278   Lyme disease (and pets)

M

235   Mad cow disease

279   Matches (and pets)

33   Medications

280   Medications (and pets)

53   Metformin

55   Methadone

170   Methanol

54   Methylphenidate

85   Mistletoe

86   Monkshood

55   Morphine

88   Morning glory

144   Mosquito bite

89   Mother-in-law plant

171   Mouthwash

101   Mushrooms

N

55 Narcotics

90 Narcissus

91 Nightshade, black

92 Nightshade, deadly

O

60 Oil of wintergreen

93 Oleander

281 Onions (and pets)

55 Opioids

174 Organochlorines

175 Organophosphates

166 Oven cleaner

55 Oxycodone

P

253 Paint (lead-based)

172 Paint (oil-based)

170 Paint remover

173 Paint thinner

177 Paraquat

60 Pennyroyal

173 Perfumes

173 Pesticides

282 Pesticides (and pets)

94 Philodendron

63 Plants, poisonous

178 Playground equipment

95 Poison ivy

95 Poison oak

95 Poison sumac

178 Pressure-treated wood

176 Pyrethrins and synthetic pyrethroids

R

180 Radon

176 Rat poison

283 Raisins (and pets)

116 Rattlesnake bite

66 Rhododendron

98 Rhubarb

54 Ritalin

S

237 Salmonellosis

60 Sassafras

151 Scorpion sting

190 Sea anemone sting

191 Sea urchin sting

170 Shellac

238 Shellfish poisoning

241 Shigellosis

114 Snakebite

148 Spider bite

242 Staphylococcal food poisoning

192 Stingray sting

182 Swimming pool cleaner

T

262 Talcum powder

56 Thyroid medication

140 Tick bite

122 Toad, poisonous

183 Toilet bowl cleaner

99 Tomato plant

243 Toxoplasmosis

244 Trichinellosis

V

246 Vibrio

W

126 Wasp sting

193 Water moccasin bite

177 Weed killer

183 Windshield washer solution

X

284 Xylitol (and pets)

Y

100 Yew

Z

176 Zinc phosphide

INTRODUCTION

A BOOK FOR EVERY HOUSEHOLD

To a toddler, the world is an endlessly fascinating place, full of things to touch and taste. Unfortunately, all too many of these things are toxic. Most of us know enough to lock up the medicines and the rat poison—but too many conscientious parents don't realize how toxic items in our environment can be. You may not realize that more than 90 percent of all accidental poisonings occur in and around the home, and 57 percent of them happen to children under age 5, from exposure to hazardous cleaning substances, plants, pesticides, cosmetics, and art supplies.

Art supplies? Yes. Even children's toys can be hazardous if you don't know what you are buying. There are many harmful substances around the house that will come as a surprise to many parents when they see them in this book. Did you know, for example, that:

✖ Ingesting a single pill for diabetes can kill a toddler?

✖ Certain species of common caterpillars can cause a harmful sting?

✖ One swallow of windshield wiper fluid can cause blindness?

✖ A child can go into seizures after eating innocent-looking mushrooms growing near home?

✖ Nibbling a poinsettia won't kill a child, but taking a bite of a rhododendron plant can lead to swelling of airways and breathing problems?

From chemicals to insecticides, from auto products to medications, every household in America can be a dangerous place for small children. How easy it is for a distracted parent to carelessly leave a bottle of pretty-colored pills half-opened on a table, or forget to close a cabinet filled with harmful cleaning products within reach of inquisitive fingers.

Medicines and chemicals are the obvious but not the only potential problems. Improperly stored or cooked food and beverages can make members of the household just as sick as a bite or sting from any toxic creature.

It is every adult's responsibility to learn what is potentially toxic in the home, and then take every precaution to keep those things locked up, out of reach and out of sight of small children. Obviously, we can't wrap our families in cotton wool and protect them from every possible danger. But the more we know about what can cause potential harm indoors and out, the more precautions we can take to make our homes, our neighborhoods, and our communities safer.

This book offers a detailed discussion of all the poisons that can be found in and around the home. You'll learn symptoms to look for, smart preventive advice, and actions to take should an accident happen. There is a desperate need for this kind of information. When the federal government established a national poison control hotline number, 44,000 people called with questions about possible poisoning within the first month. Every year, more than 2 million Americans call to report accidental poisonings.

Even though poison control center hotlines are helpful, what families really need is a handy, reliable, and informative guide that helps families both prevent and treat a problem. If you know that deicer is poisonous, you won't have to wait until your child swallows some and gets sick before taking action. If you know that the saddleback caterpillar delivers a devastating sting, you'll be able to recognize potential danger when you spot the bright green bug in your backyard. It's also a good idea that at least one person in every household be trained in lifesaving first aid and CPR, which can help you respond to poisoning and other emergencies more effectively.

Should an accident happen, remember to stay calm and call the regional Poison Control Center (1-800-222-1222) right away, and do not make the problem any worse by giving inappropriate treatments. Prompt treatment is vital, and minutes can mean the difference between life and death. First aid procedures differ according to the kind of poison involved, a child's weight, and how long the poison has been active in the body. Only medical personnel can determine the correct treatment. Treating someone without expert advice could cause further harm.

This is not a book that you buy and leave on the shelf until an accident happens. Read it and become familiar with the potential dangers in your family environment. Keep it in a handy place... just in case.

1

POISONING BASICS

FIRST AID AND PREVENTION

Sarah was a careful mom who always locked up the roach spray, rat poison, and lye. But she never realized that other household items could be just as deadly to her toddlers, including the iron in her multivitamin tablet, the furniture polish she stashed under the sink in an unlocked cupboard, the windshield washer fluid in the garage, and the colorful—and enticing—mouthwash she kept in the bathroom cabinet.

Like Sarah and most other parents, you probably think of your home as a safe haven in an unsafe world. But did you know that more than 90 percent of all poisoning accidents occur at home? And that 57 percent of poison exposures affecting kids under age 5 involve nonmedicinal substances such as cleaning products, plants, pesticides, cosmetics, and art supplies? That's why it is every adult's responsibility to learn the facts about potentially toxic products in the household and then take every precaution to keep those things either locked up or out of reach and out of sight of children.

Most poisonings occur when parents aren't paying attention or watching children as closely as they should. In fact, calls to poison control centers peak in late afternoon and early evening, because that's when busy moms and dads are trying to put dinner on the table and get chores done around the house. Poison control centers handle one poisoning case every 13 seconds— but with a little bit of forethought on your part, you can significantly increase the odds that your family won't be one of them.

Sometimes, however, despite our best efforts, a child will get into a harmful substance. In cases like these, it's important to stay calm and gather the information necessary to help your child.

IF YOU SUSPECT POISONING

If you find your child playing with or eating a household product, medicine, or plant, and you're not sure if a poisoning accident has occurred, observe your child's behavior. Remember that reactions vary depending on the product, but often a toxic substance can make your child vomit or appear drowsy or sluggish. Some of the substance may remain around the child's mouth or teeth. There may be burns around the lips or mouth from corrosive items, or you may be able to smell the product on the child's breath. However, keep in mind that some products cause no immediate symptoms.

IF YOUR CHILD HAS SWALLOWED A POISONOUS SUBSTANCE

Take the substance away from your child immediately.

Make your child spit the substance out (if possible) or remove it carefully with your fingers. Keep the material as evidence of what has been swallowed.

If your child is unconscious, not breathing, or having convulsions or seizures, call **911** or your local emergency number right away.

If your child doesn't have these symptoms, call the regional Poison Control Center hotline at **1-800-222-1222.**

Do not make your child vomit unless instructed to do so.

Do not follow instructions on packaging about poison treatment instead of calling Poison Control; package information may be outdated.

The Poison Control Center

If your child is conscious and still able to breathe without problems after a potential poisoning emergency, the regional Poison Control Center hotline (1-800-222-1222) can provide you with further instructions. This is a national toll-free number that works from anywhere in the United States, 24 hours a day, seven days a week. Keep the number by your phone—it will connect you to the closest regional Poison Control Center. There are currently more than 60 such centers in the United States that maintain information for doctors and the public on recommended treatment for the ingestion of household products and medicines. (A state-by-state list of phone numbers begins on page 288.) Poison Control Center staffers are familiar with the toxicity of most substances found in the home or know how to find this information. Follow their instructions precisely. If you can't call a control center, call 911, the operator, or your pediatrician.

Often, calling a center simply reassures you that the product your child got into isn't poisonous. In other cases, following phone instructions may help you avoid a trip to a hospital emergency room. Nearly 90 percent of callers to poison centers are told that it's safe not to seek medical care.

WHEN YOU CALL POISON CONTROL

Remain calm! Not all medicines and household chemicals are poisonous. When you contact the Poison Control Center or emergency personnel, have the substance's label or description in hand so you can provide details about the substance's contents. Be prepared to give the following information:

✗ Your child's age and weight.

✗ Existing health conditions or problems.

✗ A description of the substance and whether it was swallowed, inhaled, absorbed through skin contact, or splashed into the eyes.

✗ How long ago the poisoning occurred.

✗ Any first aid that may have been given.

✗ If your child has vomited.

✗ Your location and how long it will take you to get to the hospital.

POISONING FIRST AID

If your child has been exposed to a toxic substance, there are some immediate first aid actions you can take at home.

On the skin. If your child spills a chemical or toxic substance on the skin, call Poison Control and remove the child's clothes right away. Rinse the skin with cool or lukewarm (not hot) water. If the skin looks burned, continue rinsing for at least five minutes, even if your child may fuss. Don't use ointments, butter, or grease on the burns.

In the eye. A toxic substance may inadvertently be sprayed into your child's eyes. If this happens, flush the eye. First, hold the eyelids open; then pour a stream of lukewarm water from a container onto the bridge of the nose so it will drain across the inner corner of the eye. (Bottled saline used to rinse contact lenses also may be used.) You may need someone to help you hold the child while you rinse the eye. Continue flushing the eye for 15 minutes and then call the Poison Control Center for further instructions. Don't use an eyecup, eye drops, or eye ointment unless the poison center tells you that it's okay.

Inhaled toxic fumes or gases. In the home, your child might inhale toxic fumes by breathing in exhaust from a car running in a closed garage; vapors caused by mixing bleach and ammonia together while cleaning; fumes from solvents; leaky gas vents; or a wood, coal, or kerosene stove that isn't working properly.

These fumes or gases can overcome a person quickly, so get the child into fresh air immediately. After removing the child from danger, if she is still able to breathe without problems, call the poison center for further instructions. Even if she seems perfectly fine, get medical advice.

If your child is having trouble breathing, call 911 or your local emergency service. If your child has stopped breathing, start CPR and don't stop until your child is able to breathe again or until someone else takes over. If you can, have someone call 911 right away. If you're alone, perform CPR for one minute and then call 911.

Swallowed poison. Check and monitor your child's breathing and heartbeat. If necessary, begin rescue breathing (mouth-to-mouth resuscitation) or CPR. If possible, identify the poison and call the Poison Control Center or a physician.

Don't give your child anything to eat or drink before calling and don't induce vomiting unless a doctor or the Poison Control Center tells you to do so. Don't try to neutralize the poison with lemon juice or vinegar—or anything else—unless you're told to do so by the poison center. And don't use any "cure-all" type of antidote.

Reassure your child and keep him comfortable. If he is drowsy, position him on his left side while awaiting medical help.

Activated Charcoal: Yes or No?

Some medical experts recommend that parents should keep activated charcoal on hand in case of an accidental poisoning. When swallowed, activated charcoal latches onto poison, preventing it from being absorbed from the intestinal tract. Activated charcoal is usually sold in liquid form in 30-gram doses. You may have to ask your druggist for it, because it may not be on store shelves.

However, many experts don't think activated charcoal should be administered at home. The U.S. Consumer Product Safety Commission, for example, doesn't recommend that parents use activated charcoal because young children don't find it palatable and often refuse to drink it. The American Academy of Pediatrics (AAP) has stated that it's premature to recommend the administration of activated charcoal in the home. According to the academy, there is no evidence that administering activated charcoal at home changes the poisoning outcome, and there's a chance of harm if it's given inappropriately.

Of course, if the medical expert you contact does recommend that you administer activated charcoal, you can do so. For children under 5, give one gram per every two pounds of body weight (about one teaspoon for each 10 pounds of body weight). Older children and adults may require higher doses. Activated charcoal should be given only to a person who is conscious and fully alert. Someone who is drowsy or unconscious might inhale the charcoal into the lungs, which could lead to pneumonia. In any case, remember to call your local Poison Control Center first before giving your child any at-home antidote.

Syrup of Ipecac: Throw It Out

Many homes in the United States have a bottle of syrup of ipecac in the medicine chest, so you may be surprised to learn that since the late 1990s experts stopped recommending its routine use in poisoning emergencies.

A liquid made from the *ipecacuanha* plant, syrup of ipecac has been used for many years to induce vomiting in some cases of poison or drug ingestion. However, experts began to question the benefit of forced vomiting in the treatment of poisoning, and today poison control centers rarely recommend its use. In 2003, the AAP reversed its longstanding advice that ipecac should be kept on hand in the home and instead advised it should *not* be routinely stocked in the home medicine cabinet.

The American Association of Poison Control Centers made a similar recommendation in 2004, although it left open the option of using ipecac in circumstances when medical care is not accessible. Although it seems to make sense to induce vomiting after the ingestion of a potentially poisonous substance, this approach was never proven to be effective.

The AAP also noted that poisoning deaths have dropped dramatically over the last half century because of improved vigilance. In fact, most emergency rooms have stopped using ipecac in favor of activated charcoal, even though there is no definitive evidence that activated charcoal significantly changes the outcome.

Moreover, research has shown that ipecac has been improperly administered by parents when it was not needed or could be potentially harmful, and that it has been abused by people with eating disorders such as bulimia. Abuse of ipecac can lead to heart problems and even death.

If you have ipecac at home, experts say that you should dispose of it safely by pouring it down the drain or flushing it down the toilet.

POISON PREVENTION AROUND THE HOME

The best way to avoid a poisoning emergency in the first place is to keep sources of potential danger well away from your children. With that in mind, let's take a look at some possible trouble spots around the house.

Kitchen and Laundry

These are two of the most unsafe areas in the home because most families store their household cleaning products—everything from scouring powder and drain cleaner to laundry detergent and bleach—near the kitchen sink or in the laundry room. Research shows that more than half of all families keep those cleaners and chemicals in unlocked compartments. That's double trouble because of the close proximity to stored food and beverages. A case of mistaken identity could cause a serious poisoning. To keep your kids safe, remember to:

✖ Store food and household cleaning products in separate locations and keep the latter well secured.

✖ Never transfer poisonous or caustic products to drinking glasses, soda bottles, or other food containers.

✖ Avoid buying cleaning products or household chemicals with labels showing pictures of food (such as citrus fruit on some "lemon scented" products) or those that are packaged in containers that look similar to beverage bottles. Your children could mistake these for edible food products.

✖ Never mix household cleaning and chemical products together. A poisonous gas can be created when mixing certain chemicals—especially chlorine bleach with ammonia or acidic toilet bowl cleaner.

✖ Turn on fans and open windows when using chemical products.

✖ Keep children with asthma out of the kitchen or bathroom when using strong-smelling household cleaners.

✖ Treat vitamin and mineral supplements like medicines, not food. Keep them locked up and out of reach. It's especially important to remember that supplements containing iron can be very dangerous to a child if taken incorrectly.

Bathroom

Ideally, medicines should never be stored in the bathroom. First, a bathroom's warm, moist environment tends to cause changes or deterioration of the product. Second, too many people don't lock their bathroom medicine cabinets even when they contain a host of potentially poisonous items. So, if you aren't already doing so, consider moving medications to a well-secured closet or cabinet in an adjacent area.

Also remember that "child-resistant" does not mean "child-proof." The legal definition of a "child-resistant cap" is one that takes more than five minutes for 80 percent of 5-year-olds to open. That means that 20 percent of youngsters could still get into a medicine bottle with a child-resistant cap in less than five minutes! Kids are persistent, and they can often figure out how to open these caps.

While you're moving these substances to a safer location, take time to sort through them. Old and outdated medicines should be disposed of, because some medications can become ineffective or even dangerous over time.

Remember that some mouthwashes, aftershave lotions, and colognes contain high concentrations of alcohol. Ingested in large enough amounts, they can cause drunkenness or serious poisoning, leading to coma and even death in young children.

Children are more sensitive to the toxic effects of alcohol than are adults, and it doesn't take much alcohol to produce such reactions. Fortunately, most children find the strong, bitter taste of alcohol-containing products unappealing and rarely drink more than a harmless sip.

Living Room and Family Room

Most parents are vigilant about keeping cords out of a child's reach, sharp edges on furniture covered, and breakables out of the way. Other less obvious hazards:

Houseplants are a common part of your home's decor, but if you have small children, it's important to know each plant's name and its poison potential. Although most houseplants are not poisonous, some are. To be on the safe side, keep all houseplants out of the reach of young children.

Visitors' handbags, tote bags, and diaper bags should be stored when company arrives, since they may contain medications or other dangerous products. Weekly medication containers are a special concern, because they often hold a large number of pills and usually are not child-resistant.

Used liquor glasses and cigarette butts should not be left lying around on tables. Especially if you have young children, be sure to clean up completely immediately after parties, not the next morning.

Button-shaped batteries (used in watches, cameras, and other electronic gadgets) lying around the home can cause a problem if swallowed by a young child. In order to prevent trouble, keep all batteries out of your child's reach and throw away old batteries, securely wrapped, after they've been removed from the packaging material.

Garage/Shed

This is where most families store their highly toxic substances, including antifreeze, windshield washer fluid, insecticides, herbicides, and gasoline. All of these products should be stored out of children's reach in a locked cabinet. Childproof safety latches can be purchased at the hardware store; use them on all cupboards (top and bottom). Also:

✖ Keep potential poisons in their original containers. Never use drink containers such as cups or bottles to store chemical products and pesticides.

✖ Read and follow label directions and cautions on household and chemical products before using them.

✖ When spraying pesticides and other chemicals, wear protective clothing—long-sleeve shirts, long pants, socks, shoes, and gloves—and make sure your children are not in the area or outside playing. Pesticides can be absorbed through the skin and can be extremely poisonous, so make sure your kids stay away from areas that have recently been sprayed. For information on specific chemicals and pesticides, see Chapter 6, starting on page 155.

Now that you know the basics of dealing with poison emergencies and how to prevent poisonings in each room of the house, it's time to turn to more specific situations. In the next chapter, you'll learn how to recognize symptoms of various medication poisonings, what to do at home in such an emergency, and what to expect at the hospital.

2

AVOID ACCIDENTAL OVERDOSE

MEDICATIONS AND HERBS

Marsha had just finished giving her 2-year-old a dose of flavored liquid vitamins plus iron when a fight between the family cat and dog momentarily distracted her. With her attention elsewhere, she set the vitamin bottle on the table without fastening the top. A few seconds later, she turned around to find her daughter holding the bottle in one hand, and placing the dropper in her mouth with the other. Marsha, who had always been so careful to lock up every household chemical and drug, was horrified.

It's every parent's nightmare—and it happens all too often. Every 30 seconds, a childhood poisoning occurs in the United States. And it's not just moms and dads who need to be more vigilant. Among children 4 and younger, about a third of poisonings by prescription drugs involve a grandparent's or other relative's medication. A study conducted by the American Association of Poison Control Centers found that 23 percent of the oral prescription drugs that were swallowed by children under 5 belonged to someone who didn't live with the child. The data suggest that all adults need to use child-resistant packaging and keep medicines properly secured, away from young children.

The good news is that childproof packaging has significantly decreased accidental poisonings. But all the childproofing in the world won't help if someone gets careless and leaves an open container where a child can find it.

STORAGE DOS AND DON'TS

The key to keeping your kids safe starts with you. Here's what to do.

- Never store medicine on a counter or bedside table.

- Never assume a child won't swallow a medication because it tastes bad or the tablet is too big.

- Keep pills in their original containers, and always close and put away the container as soon as you're finished.

- Always keep medicines out of your child's sight and reach.

- Always use child-resistant caps.

- Be especially careful about keeping medicine in handbags and suitcases, which a child can easily get into.

- When visiting older friends and relatives, make sure you never let your child out of your sight, or make sure the medicine in these homes is safely locked away.

MEDICINE CABINET SAFETY

Review the contents of your medicine cabinet or closet once a month, and throw out all unneeded or expired items. Pour the contents down the drain or toilet, and rinse out the container before throwing it away.

Consider buying a cabinet lock for the medicine chest if you have toddlers or older kids who like to explore.

GIVE MEDICINE SAFELY

Keeping medicine out of reach is the most important way to prevent accidental poisonings, but it's also important to know how to administer a remedy safely when needed. While most accidental poisonings occur when a child gets into a medicine cabinet on his own, it's also possible to poison a child by giving the wrong type or wrong dose of medication.

Follow medicine label directions carefully to avoid accidental overdoses. But also recognize that sometimes pharmacists make mistakes. If anything on the label directions of your child's prescription medicine seems unusual, odd, or different than a previous refill—or if the medication itself seems different—call your pharmacist right away. Do not assume a mistake is impossible.

Here are some other safety tips to keep in mind:

✖ Never give your child medicine in the dark. Many medicine bottles look alike in dim light. Turn on a light and take the time to be sure.

✖ Be sure you know your child's current weight when asking the doctor for a prescription over the phone; weight affects dosage.

⋇ Don't substitute a kitchen teaspoon for a measuring teaspoon when giving medicine.

⋇ Throw away unused medication after an illness.

⋇ Don't give a prescription medication to anyone other than the person for whom it was prescribed.

⋇ Never coax your child to take her medicine by referring to it as "candy."

⋇ Read all label information and "caution" statements.

⋇ Get into the habit of checking the level inside a bottle of liquid medicine each time you use it. That way, if your child should accidentally get into it, you'll have a rough idea of whether the bottle was previously nearly empty or nearly full. An easy way to do this is to mark the container with a waterproof pen at the level of the liquid each time you use it.

ACT FAST: AN OVERDOSE IS AN EMERGENCY

If you suspect a drug overdose and your child is unconscious, having convulsions, or has stopped breathing, call for emergency help (911) immediately. If no symptoms are evident, don't wait to see if they develop; call the regional Poison Control Center right away. Dialing 1-800-222-1222 from anywhere in the United States will direct your call automatically to your nearest poison center. Be prepared to provide as much information as possible to the center to help determine what the next course of action should be.

ACETAMINOPHEN

COMMON BRAND NAMES

Children's Tylenol
Panadol
Tempra
Tylenol

Just because over-the-counter remedies don't require a doctor's prescription doesn't mean they are harmless. Typically, this drug is not toxic except in overdose—either taken accidentally by a child, or given too often or in an incorrect dosage by mistake.

The children's form of acetaminophen (such as Tylenol) is one of the medications most commonly misused by parents. Because it's sold in so many different dosages for children, and it's been available for years, most parents feel comfortable giving acetaminophen to children for pain or fever. Studies have found, however, that sometimes parents give too much children's acetaminophen, or they give it too often.

Of the 57,516 acetaminophen overdoses reported in one recent year, 40,774 of those involved persons under the age of 19, and 35,705 were unintentional. In 120 of these cases, the overdose was fatal.

Acetaminophen became the preferred fever reducer in the 1970s after studies showed a link between aspirin and Reye's syndrome, a potentially fatal disease in children and teens. Acetaminophen is safe if used as directed, but it can damage the liver and kidneys when given in excess amounts or when combined with alcohol.

PREVENTION!

One of the biggest concerns in acetaminophen overdose is the role that parents play in selecting a dosage to give to their children. It's particularly important for parents to understand the difference in the strengths of various formulations. Extra-strength formulations of acetaminophen may contain 500 milligrams of acetaminophen per pill, whereas a children's chewable tablet may have only 80 milligrams. If you were to give your child the same number of pills or caplets of extra- or adult-strength as of child-strength acetaminophen, you could unintentionally give more than six times the correct dose.

Be careful to use only the recommended dose and don't shorten the interval between recommended doses. Be particularly aware that acetaminophen is often included in combination products, so if you give a combination cold preparation containing acetaminophen, then give a dose of Tylenol, you're giving too much.

You should always keep track of not just the amount of the medicines you give your child, but also the frequency. If pain or fever persists for more than a few days, check with your child's doctor.

SYMPTOMS OF AN OVERDOSE

An overdose at first triggers symptoms such as loss of appetite, nausea, and vomiting. Keep in mind that there are many factors that contribute to acetaminophen toxicity. If a child has pre-existing health problems, such as an impaired liver, malnutrition, or dehydration, acetaminophen can become toxic at lower doses.

Within 24 to 48 hours after the overdose, liver injury becomes evident, with pain or tenderness in the upper right area of the abdomen, signaling liver enlargement. Jaundice (a yellowing of the skin and eyes), low blood sugar, impaired consciousness, kidney failure, and abnormal blood clotting also may occur. If symptoms progress this far without treatment, there is a possibility that the overdose may be fatal.

WHAT TO DO

Acetaminophen poisoning progresses quickly, so the faster you recognize it, the better. Call the regional Poison Control Center immediately (1-800-222-1222). If your child is unconscious or not breathing, call 911 first.

AT THE HOSPITAL

Treatment started within 10 hours of the overdose offers the best chance of a good outcome. Treatment depends on how much of the drug is in the blood. If levels are elevated, then the antidote N-acetylcysteine is given. In extreme cases involving liver failure, a liver transplant may be necessary.

ANTIANXIETY DRUGS

GENERIC NAME	BRAND NAME
Alprazolam	Xanax
Buspirone	BuSpar
Chlordiazepoxide	Librax, Libritabs, Librium
Clonazepam	Klonopin
Clorazepate	Tranxene
Diazepam	Valium
Flurazepam	Dalmane
Lorazepam	Ativan
Oxazepam	Serax
Prazepam	Centrax
Temazepam	Restoril
Triazolam	Halcion
Zolpidem	Ambien

All of these drugs except *buspirone* and *zolpidem* are benzodiazepines, which are given to ease short-term anxiety and to help induce sleep. Fatalities from overdoses are rare, unless the drug is combined with other medicines or alcohol.

SYMPTOMS OF AN OVERDOSE

These drugs cause sleepiness, slowed or slurred speech, and difficulty walking or standing. Severe overdoses can cause slowed or difficult breathing, very low blood pressure, stupor, coma, and death.

WHAT TO DO

Call the regional Poison Control Center (1-800-222-1222). The staff will determine if the situation requires hospital referral. If your child is unconscious or not breathing, call 911 first.

AT THE HOSPITAL

Usually no treatment is required other than close observation. In some circumstances the child may be given flumazenil, a drug that reverses the effects of the overdose.

ANTICONVULSANT DRUGS

GENERIC NAME	BRAND NAME
Carbamazepine	Tegretol
Phenobarbitol	Luminal, Solfoton
Phenytoin	Dilantin
Sodium valproate	Depakene

Anticonvulsant drugs (also called antiepileptics) belong to a group of pharmaceuticals used to prevent seizures. They typically work by blocking sodium channels in the brain.

SYMPTOMS OF AN OVERDOSE

Symptoms of poisoning include drowsiness, nausea, vomiting, low blood pressure, altered heart rhythm, coma, and convulsions.

WHAT TO DO

Consult the regional Poison Control Center (1-800-222-1222) for up-to-date guidance and advice. If your child is unconscious or not breathing, call 911 first.

AT THE HOSPITAL

Activated charcoal can be administered if the child is conscious. Otherwise, close observation is the only treatment necessary. For mild symptoms, your child will probably be observed for about four hours and then discharged. If symptoms are moderate or persist after four hours, your child may be admitted for further observation.

ANTIDEPRESSANTS

GENERIC NAME	BRAND NAME
Selective Serotonin Reuptake Inhibitors (SSRIs)	
Fluoxetine	Prozac
Sertraline	Zoloft
Fluvoxamine	Luvox
Paroxetine	Paxil
Citalopram	Celexa
Serotonin/Norepinephrine Reuptake Inhibitors (SNRIs)	
Nefazadone	Serzone
Venlafaxine	Effexor
Tricyclics	
Amitriptyline	Elavil, Endep
Imipramine	Norfranil, Tofranil
Nortriptyline	Aventyl, Pamelor
Desipramine	Norpramin
Doxepin	Sinequan
Protriptyline	Triptil, Vivactil
Trimipramine	Surmontil
Monoamine Oxidase Inhibitors (MAOIs)	
Phenelzine	Nardil
Tranylcypromine	Parnate
Miscellaneous drugs	
Bupropion	Wellbutrin
Mirtazepine	Remeron

Antidepressant drugs are given to treat depression and anxiety, and are available in several different main classes: selective serotonin reuptake inhibitors (SSRIs), serotonin/norepinephrine reuptake inhibitors (SNRIs), tricyclics, monoamine oxidase inhibitors (MAOIs), and a group of chemically unrelated "miscellaneous" antidepressants.

Each type of antidepressant differs in its side effects, and each causes a different reaction. In general, the newer SSRIs and SNRIs are less dangerous in overdose than the tricyclics and MAOIs. All classes are available only by prescription.

SYMPTOMS OF AN OVERDOSE

Overdoses of antidepressants can cause confusion, drowsiness, low blood pressure, seizures, and coma. Tricyclics can also cause heart rhythm disturbances. MAOIs can cause severe high blood pressure and fever.

WHAT TO DO

Call the regional Poison Control Center (1-800-222-1222). The Center will advise you on whether the amount or type of drug ingested warrants a hospital visit. If your child is unconscious or not breathing, call 911 first.

AT THE HOSPITAL

Doctors will probably give activated charcoal by mouth or through a tube in the stomach. They will likely attach a heart monitor to your child and give intravenous fluids.

For very serious poisonings, life support measures and admission to the intensive care unit may be needed. Children receiving prompt treatment and good care should recover within a few days.

MEDICATIONS

ANTI-INFLAMMATORY DRUGS (NSAIDS)

GENERIC NAME	BRAND NAME
Ibuprofen	Advil, Haltran, Medipren, Motrin, Nuprin
Naproxen	Aleve, Naprosyn

Ibuprofen and naproxen belong to a category of medications called nonsteroidal anti-inflammatory drugs (NSAIDs) and are widely used to treat inflammation and pain. They are available in both nonprescription and prescription dosage forms. Because these drugs can interfere with normal blood clotting, people with peptic ulcers, sensitive stomachs, or a history of gastrointestinal bleeding should avoid NSAIDs unless specifically directed to use them by a doctor.

SYMPTOMS OF AN OVERDOSE

A small overdose of nonprescription-strength ibuprofen or naproxen usually causes little more than stomach pain or nausea and vomiting, but massive amounts can lead to breathing problems, kidney damage, shock, and coma.

WHAT TO DO

If you suspect an overdose, call the regional Poison Control Center (1-800-222-1222); the staff will determine whether the dose taken is enough to warrant hospital evaluation.

AT THE HOSPITAL

The doctor may administer activated charcoal by mouth to bind the drug in the stomach, and may order blood tests to check for any kidney problems.

ASPIRIN

GENERIC NAME	BRAND NAME
Aspirin	Ascriptin
	Aspergum
	Bayer Aspirin
	Bufferin
	Children's Bayer Aspirin
	Ecotrin
	Empirin

This common painkiller was used much more often in the past, and at one time was routinely given to children for fever and pain. Today the incidence of aspirin poisoning is decreasing, in part because of child-resistant packaging, but also because so many families no longer use aspirin.

In the 1970s, studies showed a link between aspirin use for influenza or chickenpox and Reye's syndrome, a potentially fatal disease that attacks the internal organs of children under the age of 18. As a result, pediatricians no longer recommend giving aspirin to children.

Nevertheless, there are a number of ways that aspirin poisoning can occur, since more than 200 different products contain aspirin. Salicylates (the active ingredient in aspirin) are also found in many medicated skin creams. Once on the skin, they can be absorbed, leading to poisoning in children.

SYMPTOMS OF AN OVERDOSE

In large doses, aspirin stimulates the central nervous system, causing rapid breathing, confusion, and convulsions. Similar symptoms can occur in people who are allergic to aspirin. Other symptoms include abdominal pain, fever, nausea, vomiting, dehydration, restlessness, coma, and respiratory failure.

WHAT TO DO

If you suspect an overdose, call the regional Poison Control Center (1-800-222-1222) immediately. The staff at the poison center will determine if the exposure was serious enough to warrant a visit to the emergency room.

AT THE HOSPITAL

Doctors may administer activated charcoal orally to adsorb any remaining aspirin in the digestive tract. Activated charcoal is most effective if given soon after the overdose. However, it still may be useful even in children who get to the hospital hours after the overdose. The challenge is to give activated charcoal despite the child's nausea and vomiting.

Doctors will do blood tests to determine the severity of poisoning, and may give intravenous fluids. For very severe cases, hemodialysis may be needed to remove aspirin from the blood.

BIRTH CONTROL PILLS

Birth control pills—medications containing the hormones progesterone or estrogen, or their derivatives—are not considered to be toxic when ingested accidentally by children, although they may cause nausea and vomiting.

BLOOD PRESSURE MEDICATION

GENERIC NAME	BRAND NAME
Clonidine	Catapres

Clonidine is a medication used to treat high blood pressure. As little as 0.1 milligram of clonidine has produced signs of toxicity in children. Accidental overdose of clonidine is an increasing cause of poisoning in children 3 and under.

SYMPTOMS OF AN OVERDOSE

Clonidine ingestion may cause slowed heart rate, depression of the central nervous system, low body temperature, abnormal heart rhythms, weakened reflexes, sleepiness, nausea, vomiting, or constricted pupils.

WHAT TO DO

Consult the regional Poison Control Center (1-800-222-1222) for up-to-date guidance and advice. If your child is unconscious or not breathing, call 911 first.

AT THE HOSPITAL

Aggressive cardiovascular treatment is necessary for managing these types of overdoses, depending on the symptoms, and your child's blood pressure and heart rate will be monitored. Activated charcoal may be given.

COLD MEDICATIONS

Drugstore and grocery shelves are filled with a wide variety of every type of cold preparation aimed at relieving a child's sneezing, sniffling, coughing, and fever. It's no wonder that almost every family with young children has a few bottles of over-the-counter children's cold medication stashed away in the medicine cabinet. Yet pediatricians worry that parents may not realize how easy it is to give a child an overdose by combining common cold and fever medications.

Of biggest concern is the real possibility of giving an overdose of fever reducers, which can affect the liver or the kidneys. Some children's cough and cold medications, such as Dimetapp and

MEDICATIONS

Triaminic, contain fever-reducing acetaminophen or ibuprofen. Because some parents may not realize this, they give their children cold medicine plus an extra fever-reducing medication such as Tylenol (acetaminophen) or Motrin/Advil (ibuprofen), resulting in an overdose. Other ingredients in cough and cold preparations that can cause problems when given in excess include:

✖ Antihistamines: brompheniramine, chlorpheniramine, diphenhydramine, and doxylamine

✖ Decongestant: pseudoephedrine

✖ Cough suppressant: dextromethorphan

PREVENTION!
Before you give any medication to your child, check the label to see what the active ingredients are and compare these with other drugs the child is already taking. If the same active ingredient is found in more than one product, don't use both.

SYMPTOMS OF AN OVERDOSE
Depending on the specific ingredients, symptoms of overdose with a cough or cold product may include dry mouth, enlarged pupils, flushing, sweating, rapid heartbeat, hyperactivity or agitation, hallucinations, stumbling or loss of coordination, seizures, or coma.

WHAT TO DO
Call the regional Poison Control Center (1-800-222-1222). If your child is unconscious or not breathing, call 911 first.

AT THE HOSPITAL
Doctors may administer activated charcoal to bind the drug in the stomach, and will provide treatment for specific symptoms if they occur. If the cold medication taken contains acetaminophen, they will do a blood test to determine if the antidote N-acetylcysteine is needed.

HEART MEDICATIONS

GENERIC NAME	BRAND NAME
Beta blockers	
Acebutolol	Sectra
Atenolol	Tenormin
Betaxolol	Kerlone
Bisoprolol	Zebeta
Carteolol	Cartrol
Esmolol	Brevibloc
Labetalol	Normodyne, Trandate
Metoprolol	Toprol XL, Lopressor
Nadolol	Corgard
Penbutolol	Levatol
Pindolol	Visken
Propranolol	Inderal
Sotalol	Betapace, Sotacor
Timolol	Blocadren
Calcium channel blockers	
Felodipine	Plendil
Nifedipine	Adalat, Adalat C, Procardia, Procardia XL
Diltiazem	Cardizem, Cartia, Dilacor, Tiazac
Nicardipine	Cardene
Verapamil	Calan, Covera, Isoptin, Verelan
Digoxin	Lanoxin

A major source of childhood poisonings is the large variety of drugs prescribed to treat heart problems. Beta blockers are given to slow the heart rate and reduce the force of the heart muscle's contraction. They are used to treat high blood pressure, arrhythmias, angina, migraines, and glaucoma.

Calcium channel blockers were introduced for use in the United States in 1981 to treat chest pain, high blood pressure, arrhythmias, and migraines. Today, calcium channel blocker overdose is quickly emerging as the most lethal prescription drug overdose. In 2002, the American Association of Poison Control Centers (APCC) reported 9,585 exposures to calcium channel blockers, resulting in 68 fatalities and 365 serious illnesses; 24 percent occurred in children under age 6.

Digoxin (Lanoxin) is used to regulate the heart's rhythm after congestive heart failure, increasing contractions and reducing fluid retention.

SYMPTOMS OF AN OVERDOSE

The response to an overdose of beta blockers varies, depending on overall health and whether or not the child has asthma. Symptoms may include confusion, sweating, breathing problems and wheezing, irregular heartbeat, low blood pressure, shock, coma, and convulsions. For some children, even a normal adult dose can be fatal.

Symptoms of calcium channel blocker overdose include slowed heart rate and low blood pressure. In young children, fatal overdoses can occur with as little as one tablet.

Symptoms of digoxin overdose include nausea and vomiting, diarrhea, blurred vision, and heart problems.

WHAT TO DO

Consult the regional Poison Control Center (1-800-222-1222) for up-to-date guidance and advice. If your child is unconscious or not breathing, call 911 first. Heart medications are dangerous to children and can be fatal. Immediate action is necessary.

AT THE HOSPITAL

Most overdoses require hospitalization. Aggressive cardiovascular treatment is necessary for managing these types of overdoses, depending on the symptoms, and your child's blood pressure and heart rate will be monitored. Activated charcoal may be given.

IRON IN DRUGS AND SUPPLEMENTS

✖ Ferrous fumarate

✖ Ferrous gluconate

✖ Ferrous sulfate

Just about every family has at least one bottle of multivitamins or other supplements containing iron stashed away in the kitchen or bathroom cabinet. Even children's vitamins often contain iron, yet many parents don't realize how deadly an overdose of this mineral can be.

Supplemental iron (listed as either ferrous fumarate, ferrous gluconate, or ferrous sulfate) is commonly given to children as part of a daily multivitamin. Since 1986, more than 11,000 poisoning incidents involving children ingesting iron have been reported, and 35 children have died. Most of the serious poisonings occurred as a result of children swallowing adult-strength products containing more than 30 milligrams of iron per pill. This includes most prenatal vitamins, which are likely to be found in households with young children. Children's chewable vitamins with iron rarely cause a problem, as they contain smaller amounts of iron and are less irritating to the stomach.

Young children have been seriously injured by swallowing doses of 200 milligrams to 400 milligrams of iron, equivalent to fewer than 10 tablets of a typical adult iron supplement. An accidental overdose of iron can damage the stomach, liver, and small intestine, and lower the blood pressure, leading to shock and death.

Since 1997, all medications and supplements containing iron must display a warning about accidental overdose. Products containing 30 milligrams or more of iron per unit must be packaged as individual doses, thus limiting the number of pills a small child could swallow. This packaging change alone has resulted in a decreased incidence of death from iron overdose in children. The number of reported pediatric deaths from iron overdose went from 11 in 1991 to 0 in 2001.

PREVENTION!

The danger is still real. Be vigilant by taking three simple steps to protect your kids from this medication risk:

✖ Reclose the child-resistant package of iron-containing supplements immediately after use—every time.

✖ Keep the product out of the reach of children, preferably locked in a medicine closet or cabinet—always.

SYMPTOMS OF AN OVERDOSE

Symptoms will usually appear within 30 minutes of overdose, and include vomiting (sometimes bloody), diarrhea, and lethargy. Children with serious poisonings often have a fast weak pulse, low blood pressure, and pallor, and may go into a coma.

WHAT TO DO

Call the regional Poison Control Center (1-800-222-1222). Iron poisoning isn't something you can treat on your own. If your child is unconscious or not breathing, call 911 first.

AT THE HOSPITAL

If the poison center personnel determines that the amount ingested could cause a serious problem, they may direct the physician to obtain X-rays to look for the pills in the stomach. If pills are seen, a procedure called whole bowel irrigation may be needed. In this procedure, large amounts of a specially formulated gut-cleansing solution are given by mouth or through a tube placed into the stomach, washing the contents down the intestinal tract until they are expelled. Blood samples will probably be taken to check the amount of iron in the blood. For children with serious signs of iron poisoning, intravenous fluids and chelating agents (which bind the iron and remove it from the bloodstream) may be needed.

ISONIAZID

BRAND NAME
Lanizid
Nydrazid

This antimicrobial medication is used to treat tuberculosis, an infection that primarily affects the lungs. Tuberculosis may seem uncommon in the United States today, but poisoning with isoniazid is not uncommon.

SYMPTOMS OF AN OVERDOSE
Symptoms typically appear within 30 to 45 minutes of ingestion, and include nausea and vomiting, vague abdominal pain, irritability, lethargy, confusion, and seizures.

WHAT TO DO
Consult the regional Poison Control Center (1-800-222-1222) for up-to-date guidance and advice. If your child is unconscious or not breathing, call 911 first.

AT THE HOSPITAL
Activated charcoal may be administered as soon as possible, preferably within two hours of ingestion. Symptoms will be treated, and health professionals will check for changes in breathing

and blood pressure. If seizure and/or lethargy occur, your child may be given pyridoxine (vitamin B6) to counteract the effects of the drug.

METFORMIN

BRAND NAME
Glucomet

Glucophage

This drug is given to improve the way the body handles glucose in people with type 2 diabetes. It also lowers levels of cholesterol, triglycerides, and other fats. It is typically prescribed to people with diabetes who don't need to take insulin, but who have trouble controlling their disease through diet alone.

SYMPTOMS OF AN OVERDOSE
Children may develop vomiting, diarrhea, or drowsiness. Although rare, lethargy and coma have been reported. In rare cases, overdose can lead to a serious complication called lactic acidosis, which is a buildup of lactic acid in the blood.

WHAT TO DO
Consult the regional Poison Control Center (1-800-222-1222) for up-to-date guidance and advice. If your child is unconscious or not breathing, call 911 first.

AT THE HOSPITAL
Activated charcoal may be administered within an hour of ingestion. Otherwise, symptoms are treated as they appear. Arterial blood gases, electrolytes and blood levels of lactate may be monitored. In severe cases, hemodialysis may be necessary to remove metformin from the blood and to correct acidosis (an abnormal increase in the acidity of the body's fluids).

METHYLPHENIDATE

BRAND NAME
Ritalin

Ritalin is a common mild central nervous system stimulant pre-scribed for thousands of American children for the treatment of attention deficit hyperactivity disorder (ADHD), attention deficit disorder (ADD), and other psychological, educational, and social disorders. It is also used to treat narcolepsy, a disorder involving uncontrollable brief sleeping spells, and mild depression in the elderly.

SYMPTOMS OF AN OVERDOSE

In overdose, Ritalin can overstimulate the central nervous system and cause agitation, tremors, muscle twitching, convulsions, euphoria, confusion, hallucinations, delirium, sweating, flushing, headache, fever, rapid heart rate, palpitations, heart arrhythmias, high blood pressure, and dryness of mucous membranes. There is some evidence that prolonged use can lead to an addiction.

WHAT TO DO

Consult the regional Poison Control Center (1-800-222-1222) for up-to-date guidance and advice. If your child is unconscious or not breathing, call 911 first.

AT THE HOSPITAL

Doctors will take appropriate action to treat symptoms. Your child's blood pressure and heart rate will be monitored. Activated charcoal, which binds with the drug and removes it from the sys-tem, may be administered by mouth or by a stomach tube. Intravenous fluids and medicines may be given to normalize blood pressure or treat agitation or seizures.

OPIOIDS (NARCOTICS)

GENERIC NAME	BRAND NAME
Codeine	Codeine
Fentanyl	Acti, Duragesic
Hydrocodone	Anexsia, Lorcet, Norca, Vicodin
Hydromorphone	Dilaudid
Methadone	Dolophine
Morphine	Astramorph
Oxycodone	OxyContin
Propoxyphene	Darvon

MEDICATIONS

These narcotic painkillers, initially derived from the poppy plant, are found in numerous products, such as cough suppressants and other painkillers. Supertoxic, these medications are used to treat moderate to severe pain and can be found in combination with a wide range of other drugs, such as acetaminophen, aspirin, caffeine, and cough suppressants. In fact, more than 40 cough medicines still contain codeine.

SYMPTOMS OF AN OVERDOSE

Within minutes of ingestion, your child may start to feel sleepy, giddy, and clumsy; heartbeat slows. This can lead to breathing problems, coma, and death. Liquid forms of the drugs may cause poisoning even faster.

WHAT TO DO

Consult the regional Poison Control Center (1-800-222-1222) for up-to-date guidance and advice. If your child is unconscious or not breathing, call 911 first.

AT THE HOSPITAL

Symptoms will be treated, including monitoring of your child's blood pressure and heart rate. The antidote naloxone may be given to counteract the effects of the narcotic.

THYROID MEDICATION

GENERIC NAME	BRAND NAME
Levothyroxine	Levothroid, Synthroid
Liothyronine	Cytome
Liotrix	Thyrolar

Thyroid medication is given to balance an incorrect level of thyroid hormone in the body (either too much or too little). Toxicity is rare. If proper treatment is received quickly, recovery from thyroid medication poisoning is very likely—unless there are heart-related complications, which may be in fatal.

SYMPTOMS OF AN OVERDOSE

Symptoms are not necessarily associated with the degree of toxicity. They can include diarrhea, irregular heartbeat, headache, tremors, nervousness, stomach cramps, fever, chest pain, or difficulty sleeping.

WHAT TO DO

Consult the regional Poison Control Center (1-800-222-1222) for up-to-date guidance and advice.

AT THE HOSPITAL

Activated charcoal may be administered, and symptoms will be treated. Blood tests may be given to measure levels of thyroid hormone.

HERBAL PRODUCTS

Herbal medicine appeals to consumers who believe that herbs are better and less dangerous than synthetic drugs. However, just because a remedy is "natural" doesn't mean it's safe. A number of herbal products commonly sold can be poisonous to children and adults.

Most medicinal herbs have a long folk history, but there are some that never have been scientifically tested for their medicinal value or safety in adults, much less children. Since Americans spend billions of dollars on herbal supplements each year, odds are that at least some of them are given to children.

Though herbal products are widely available, they are only minimally regulated by the U.S. Food and Drug Administration (FDA), meaning labels can make unsubstantiated claims. This means an herbal product can contain an overdose of an active ingredient or no active ingredient at all. Moreover, herbal remedies are often marketed on the Internet with misleading and unproven claims. Manufacturers can legally call a product by its plant name, even if it contains only a tiny quantity of the herb. Most products available on health food store shelves have not been checked by any government agency for contents or potency.

Moreover, herbs can be contaminated with toxic heavy metals such as lead or mercury. There is also evidence that some herbal products imported from China may be doctored with steroids, pharmaceutical products, or other dangerous substances. In 1994, the U.S. Congress passed legislation that dramatically changed how herbal products were viewed by the government. This act, titled the Dietary Supplement Health and Education Act (DSHEA), classified dietary supplements as foods, exempting them from the same safety standards to which prescription drugs and over-the-counter medications must adhere. Herbal products, however, have biological and chemical properties that can cause potentially harmful health effects, either when used alone or in combination with pharmaceutical medicines.

There are an estimated 29,000 dietary supplements on the market, with another 1,000 new products introduced each year, according to the Institute of Medicine. During a six-month period in 2004, the FDA inspected 180 domestic dietary supplement manufacturers, sent 119 warning letters to dietary supplement distributors, refused entry to 1,171 foreign shipments of dietary supplements, and seized or supervised voluntary destruction of almost $18 million worth of mislabeled or adulterated products.

In 1998, the American Association of Poison Control Centers received four reports of children under age 6 developing life-threatening complications after taking dietary supplements (not including vitamins and minerals). Another 192 youngsters had less serious reactions.

PREVENTION!

If you're intent on taking herbal products, it's best to select well-known brands manufactured in developed countries (especially the United States and Germany) to reduce the risk of contamination. When possible, choose a product that has been "standardized" (you'll see this term on the label). Standardized herb products have been manufactured according to European standards; their labels list the amount of herb per dose and the percentage of its active ingredient. Herbs that are potentially dangerous should be avoided no matter where they are produced. They include:

- ✖ Chaparral

- ✖ Comfrey (*symphytum officinale, uplandicum,* and *asperum*)

- ✖ Eucalyptus oil

- ✖ Ephedra, or ma-huang (*ephedra sinica*)

- ✖ Germander (*teucrium chamaedrys*)

- ✖ Kava (*piper methysticum*)

- ✖ Oil of wintergreen (methyl salicylate)

- ✖ Pennyroyal (*mentha pulegium*)

- ✖ Sassafras (*sassafras albidum*)

Chaparral

Available as a tea, tablets, or capsules, chaparral is usually prepared from the leaflets and twigs of the plant. It is currently promoted as an antioxidant or "free radical scavenger" and used to treat a variety of skin conditions, such as acne. Long-term ingestion of chaparral has been associated with liver damage and possibly kidney disease.

Comfrey

Once quite popular, comfrey tea was traditionally used to treat wounds, sprains, and broken bones. The roots and leaves of this herb contain allantoin, a substance purported to help heal wounds and regenerate tissue. However, during the 1980s experts began to realize that comfrey tea could be poisonous. Research revealed that comfrey contains dangerous substances (pyrrolizidine alkaloids) that can cause severe liver damage. Children should never be given comfrey tea or products containing comfrey. Because there hasn't been any research on the pediatric use of comfrey ointments or creams, they are not recommended for children.

Eucalyptus oil

This herbal oil is often used in vaporizers and as an ointment for younger children with chest colds. However, the oil can be poisonous if swallowed. As little as 1 milliliter of eucalyptus oil has caused coma in a child and 5 milliliters has been fatal. All vaporizer fluids should be kept out of reach of young children, preferably in a child-resistant cupboard.

Ephedra, or ma-huang

Diet pills and over-the-counter medications containing the stimulant ephedra can be dangerous, causing agitation, high blood pressure, rapid heartbeat, and convulsions. In April 2004, a federal judge upheld the government's ban on the supplement. Before imposing the ban, the FDA logged almost 17,000 adverse health reactions to ephedra, including strokes, seizures, and deaths.

Germander

Marketed as a weight-loss substance, this herb can cause liver inflammation and damage, and occasionally death.

Kava

Sold as a sedative, muscle relaxant, anticonvulsant, and anti-anxiety remedy, kava has been associated with liver failure.

Oil of wintergreen

Originally derived from the wintergreen plant, oil of wintergreen is now commonly found in liniments, lotions, creams, and ointments for the treatment of muscle and joint pain. Because oil of wintergreen is almost 100 percent methyl salicylate, one teaspoonful is equivalent to about 21 adult-strength aspirin tablets. Just one swallow of oil of wintergreen can be lethal to a young child.

Because it's a concentrated liquid that is absorbed rapidly, oil of wintergreen poses a threat of severe, rapid-onset poisoning. Ingestion can cause breathing problems, dehydration, ringing in the ears, lethargy, nausea, vomiting, seizures, low blood pressure, coma, and death.

Pennyroyal

An herb traditionally used to induce abortions, pennyroyal can cause liver damage and a profound drop in blood sugar. The concentrated oil is especially poisonous, and can cause convulsions, shock, and organ failure. There are reports of fatalities in young children given pennyroyal tea.

Sassafras

The bark of this herb was once used to produce the flavor of root beer. It comes from a large tree believed to be native to Florida. The oil of the sassafras tree is volatile, and a child who drinks the oil may experience nausea, vomiting, dizziness, and hallucinations.

FOLK REMEDIES

Some Hispanic, Asian, Middle Eastern, and Native American folk medicine practices consider heavy metals such as lead to be therapeutic. Certain folk remedies for digestive ailments have been found to contain very high lead levels. These include Azarcon, Alarcon, Coral, Pay-loo-ah, and Greta. The products often come in the form of a capsule or a yellow-orange powder. Avoid them.

3

LET THEM BE

TOXIC PLANTS, SHRUBS, TREES, AND MUSHROOMS

Before a newborn infant is even brought home from the hospital, every parent should understand which houseplants are safe and which are not. And because infants turn into inquisitive toddlers in the blink of an eye, you need to know as much as possible about toxic plants, shrubs, trees, and mushrooms your child might encounter outdoors as well.

Fortunately, few plants are significantly toxic if simply tasted by a child. Most severe plant poisonings involving children occur when an adult unknowingly feeds them misidentified foraged plants. Still, each year more than 100,000 exposures to toxic plants are reported to poison centers around the country. Most of these exposures are not terribly serious because kids are usually caught before they eat too much.

Typically, how much of the plant your child eats affects the length of time before symptoms appear; the more the child swallows, the quicker the effects. For nearly all plants, your response to a potential poisoning should be the same: If you suspect your child has swallowed a poisonous plant, you should call the regional Poison Control Center (1-800-222-1222) immediately. The staff will determine if the exposure was serious enough to warrant a visit to the hospital, and they can put you in direct contact with 911 if necessary. Don't administer anything by mouth unless directed to do so by the poison center.

In almost all cases of plant poisoning, if the child gets to the hospital or the doctor's office within the first hour, can safely swallow, and isn't constantly vomiting, the health-care provider can administer activated charcoal to help bind the toxin before it's absorbed into the blood. There are very few antidotes for plant poisoning, and with a few exceptions, treatment involves observation and frequent checks on vital signs.

Intravenous fluids and electrolyte replacement may be necessary if the child has become dehydrated as a result of vomiting. If seizures develop, medications such as a benzodiazepine may be administered. If the heart rate becomes too slow, atropine may be necessary. In rare cases where the blood pressure becomes too low, medications may be administered to increase it. In the worst cases, life support using breathing machines may be necessary. Hospitals no longer induce vomiting or pump out the stomach in plant poisoning emergencies.

CHILD-SAFE PLANTS

You don't have to throw out all your houseplants or strip your grounds bare if you have small children at home—there are plenty of attractive green, growing things that are perfectly safe. Here's a list of plants you can feel comfortable having in or around the house. They are essentially nontoxic if chewed or eaten.

PLANTS

African violet	Dandelion	Prayer plant
Aluminum plant	Easter lily	Purple passion
Aspidistra	Gardenia	Rose
Aster	Impatiens	Sensitive plant
Baby's tears	Jade plant	Spider plant
Begonia	Kalanchoe	Swedish ivy
Bird's nest fern	Lipstick plant	Tiger lily
California poppy	Magnolia	Umbrella tree
Camellia	Nasturtium	Violet
Christmas cactus	Norfolk Island pine	Wandering Jew
Coleus	Pepperomia	Wax plant
Creeping charlie	Petunia	Wild strawberry
Dahlia	Poinsettia	Zebra plant

POINSETTIA: IT'S SAFE!

Although much has been made of potential harm from ingesting the foliage of the poinsettia (blamed for a poisoning death as early as 1919), recent studies indicate that this highly favored holiday houseplant is not toxic, as was once believed. At worst, eating a poinsettia leaf might cause some stomach irritation and burning in the mouth—but it`s not fatal.

AZALEA/RHODODENDRON

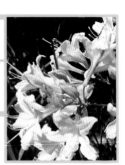

SCIENTIFIC NAME
Rhododendron

Once considered to be two separate gen-era, the azalea (pictured here) and the rho-dodendron are actually in the same genus: *Rhododendron*. The 800 species of rhododendron are subdivided into eight subgen-era. All parts of the azalea/rhododendron are toxic, containing the same poison (grayanotoxin) as in mountain laurel, which is also poisonous to eat. Honey derived purely from the nectar of azal-ea/rhododendron plants has caused mass poisonings of people who purchased the product. That's why commercial producers mix honey from several different hives to assure dilution of any potentially contaminated honey. Fortunately, most exposures result in no ill effects. However, exposure to these plants could be toxic if your child ate a large amount of an azalea/rhododen-dron plant.

SYMPTOMS OF POISONING
After chewing on the leaves, a child may experience burning in the mouth followed within six hours by nausea, vomiting, increased salivation, and abdominal pain. In the worst cases, although exceedingly rare, symptoms might include breathing problems, slowed heartbeat, low blood pressure, muscle weak-ness progressing to paralysis, convulsions, coma, and death.

WHAT TO DO
Contact the regional Poison Control Center (1-800-222-1222) immediately. The staff at the center will determine if the expo-sure was serious enough to warrant a visit to the hospital.

AT THE HOSPITAL

Children with repeated vomiting could become dehydrated. Fluid and electrolyte replacement may be necessary. In cases of severe poisoning, the drug atropine may be administered for slow heart rate, and medications such as dopamine or phenylephrine may be given for low blood pressure.

BELLADONNA   SEE NIGHTSHADE, DEADLY

CHINABERRY TREE

SCIENTIFIC NAME
Melia azedarach

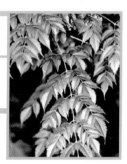

For more than 200 years this fast-growing tree has been popular in the southern United States, where it is grown for its attractive flowers and shade. In the deep South, chinaberry trees have been traditionally planted in the yard where they are thought to bring good luck. Homeowners like the showy lavender flowers in spring and the cool shade provided on hot summer days. Unfortunately, the tree easily reseeds itself, providing the homeowner with quantities of unwanted seedlings that require effort to control. As chinaberry has become established in many areas, it's turned into a pest that invades natural plant communities and displaces native species.

If that isn't bad enough, various strains of the chinaberry tree are poisonous, containing neurotoxic and potentially lethal compounds. The leaves, bark, and fruit are all potentially toxic. Birds that eat the seeds can become paralyzed. Children who eat just six to eight berries have died. The fruits are used to make insect repellent and flea powders.

SYMPTOMS OF POISONING

Ill effects may be delayed, and can include nausea, vomiting, and abdominal pain. In rare cases, poisoning can progress to lack of coordination, confusion, and faintness. More serious symptoms such as convulsions, paralysis, and even death may occur within one day of ingesting any part of this tree. A person also can be poisoned from drinking tea made from its leaves.

WHAT TO DO

If your child has ingested seeds or any part of this tree, call the regional Poison Control Center hotline (1-800-222-1222) and follow instructions. The staff at the center will determine if the exposure was serious enough to warrant a visit to the hospital. They can directly place you in contact with 911 if necessary. Do not administer anything by mouth unless directed to do so by the poison center.

AT THE HOSPITAL

If your child is seen by a doctor within the first couple of hours and does not have continuous vomiting, activated charcoal is the recommended initial treatment. Electrolyte replacement and intravenous fluids also may be necessary.

CHRISTMAS ROSE

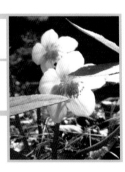

SCIENTIFIC NAME
Helleborus niger

This very poisonous relative of the buttercup family has been used medicinally since ancient times to treat mental disorders and lice. It has also been utilized as a classic poison; in Africa, for example, it was put on arrow tips. Today, it is often brought into the home by unwary parents as a Christmas decorative plant. It is found naturally in the northern United States and Canada, where it blooms from late fall through early spring, often in the snow. Its pink-white flowers appear during the Christmas season in milder climates.

The entire Christmas rose plant is toxic, but the rhizome (the thickened stem that grows horizontally below or at the soil surface) is particularly toxic. The toxins in this plant aren't destroyed by drying or storage. Although both animals and humans can be affected, poisoning with this plant is fairly rare.

SYMPTOMS OF POISONING

Following ingestion of Christmas rose, a child may experience a burning taste and blistering of the mouth, followed by slow and irregular pulse, weakness, labored breathing, irregular heartbeat, convulsions, delirium, and even death due to respiratory collapse.

WHAT TO DO

If you suspect an overdose, call the regional Poison Control Center (1-800-222-1222) immediately. The staff at the center will determine if the exposure was serious enough to warrant a visit to the hospital. Do not administer anything by mouth unless directed to do so by the poison center.

AT THE HOSPITAL

Children who have marked vomiting may experience dehydration. Fluid and electrolyte replacement may be necessary. In those cases with severe toxicity, atropine may be administered for slow heart rate, as well as dopamine or phenylephrine for low blood pressure.

CLEMATIS

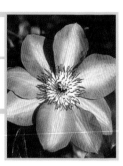

Clematis

This beautiful flowering vine—a member of the buttercup family—is grown throughout Canada and the northern temperate zone of the United States. Producing a wide variety of colorful blooms, clematis is highly prized as a perennial ornamental. Unfortunately, all parts of this plant are poisonous, and can irritate both skin and mucous membranes if eaten by a curious child. Luckily, the immediate pain caused by chewing the leaves or flowers usually causes the child to spit out the plant, limiting the amount of toxin.

SYMPTOMS OF POISONING

Soon after eating any part of this plant, a child may experience severe pain, inflammation, and blistering of the mouth, tongue, and throat, with increased salivation, stomach cramps, dizziness, and bloody diarrhea.

WHAT TO DO

If your child eats any part of this plant, call the regional Poison Control Center (1-800-222-1222) and follow instructions. The staff at the center will determine if the exposure was serious enough to warrant a visit to the hospital. The staff at the center can place you in direct contact with 911 if necessary. Do not give anything to your child by mouth unless directed to do so by the poison center.

AT THE HOSPITAL

The recommended initial treatment is administration of activated charcoal, if your child arrives within the first couple of hours and is not continuously vomiting. In rare cases, intravenous fluids and electrolyte replacement may be necessary.

CROCUS, AUTUMN

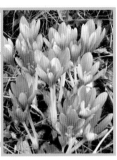

SCIENTIFIC NAMES

Colchicum autumnale
C. speciosum
C. vernum

Often mistaken for an onion, this member of the lily family has long purple or white flowers that appear from an underground bulb. It grows in damp and wooded areas. Long recognized for its toxicity, autumn crocus has been used since ancient times as a natural abortive to end pregnancy. All parts of the plant—but especially the bulb—are toxic.

The toxic substance in the plant is colchicine, found in the seeds of *C. autumnale.* Some people may be familiar with the name because a drug by the same name that is derived from the plant is used to treat gout. If goats, which are immune to the autumn crocus' toxin, eat the plant, they may pass on the poison in their milk to anyone who drinks it. Children have been poisoned by eating the flowers, and poisoning also has been reported in all types of livestock (except goats). This plant may be fatal if eaten.

SYMPTOMS OF POISONING

Within six hours of ingestion, your child may experience nausea, vomiting, bloody diarrhea, and abdominal pain. In the worst cases, those exposed may develop sensory disturbances, muscle weakness, delirium, coma, and failure of the heart, lungs, liver, and kidneys.

WHAT TO DO

If you suspect an overdose, call the regional Poison Control Center number (1-800-222-1222) immediately. Personnel at the center can determine if the exposure was serious enough to warrant a visit to the hospital. They can place you in direct contact with 911 if necessary. Do not give anything to your child by mouth unless directed to do so by the poison center.

AT THE HOSPITAL

If your child is taken to the hospital within the first couple of hours and isn't continuously vomiting, activated charcoal is likely to be administered. Electrolyte replacement and intravenous fluids may be necessary. Painkillers and atropine may be given to ease stomach pain and diarrhea. Because the toxin is excreted slowly, it can cause a slowly progressive illness that can lead to failure of many organs over a number of days. It may take weeks to recover. Death has been reported, which can occur days after ingestion. However, it is rare for a child to eat an amount large enough to cause severe illness.

DAFFODIL

SEE NARCISSUS

DEATH CAMAS

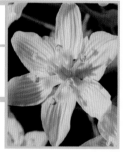

SCIENTIFIC NAME
Zigadenus venenosus

As its name implies, the death camas is highly poisonous. A lily often mistaken for an onion, and found throughout North America and Canada, this plant grows up to two feet tall, with grassy, long, and narrow leaves and a branched cluster of green, white, or yellow flowers. Fresh leaves, stems, bulbs, and flowers are all toxic, but the seeds are especially deadly. Cattle are the usual victims of death camas poisoning, but humans also can be poisoned. It is especially toxic to children.

SYMPTOMS OF POISONING

Within one hour of ingestion, a child may experience burning of the mouth, excessive thirst, vomiting, weakness, slow heartbeat, and staggering gait. If large amounts are eaten, symptoms may progress to paralysis, convulsions, coma, and death.

WHAT TO DO

If you suspect death camas poisoning, call the regional Poison Control Center (1-800-222-1222) immediately. The staff at the center will determine if the exposure was serious enough to warrant a visit to the hospital.

AT THE HOSPITAL

The recommended initial treatment is administration of activated charcoal, if your child is brought to the hospital within the first couple of hours and is not vomiting. Electrolyte replacement and intravenous fluids may be necessary. Atropine may be administered for slowed heart rate.

DUMBCANE

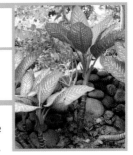

SCIENTIFIC NAME
Dieffenbachia

Dumbcane has been used as a decorative indoor plant for hundreds of years. Although it is so common we think of it as harmless, the plant can cause severe mouth pain if chewed. Ingested in large enough quantities, it can be fatal.

   Dumbcane belongs to the same family as jack-in-the-pulpit and philodendron. There are a number of different species, all of which love the shade and have large, bright green leaves. All parts of this plant are toxic, including the sap.

SYMPTOMS OF POISONING

All types of dieffenbachia contain a number of different irritants that can cause serious tissue damage to the skin, eyes, or mucous membranes. A child who gnaws on a leaf of this plant will experience almost immediate sharp, blistering, and burning pain in the mouth and on the tongue, excessive salivation, and swelling of the tongue and throat. Pain and swelling may linger for a few days.

Because of the immediate burning pain, it is unlikely that a child will eat very much of this plant at one time, so risk of a serious reaction is small. Prolonged chewing, however, could be fatal by causing the throat to swell and close, blocking the airway.

WHAT TO DO

Call the regional Poison Control Center number (1-800-222-1222) immediately. The staff at the poison center will determine if the exposure was serious enough to warrant a trip to the emergency room. The center can place you in direct contact with 911 if necessary.

AT THE HOSPITAL

In more severe cases of poisoning, antihistamines may help. In the worst cases, swelling may occur and lead to closure of the airway. In such instances, an artificial airway and life support may be necessary.

FOXGLOVE

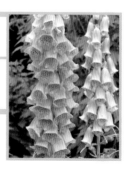

SCIENTIFIC NAME
Digitalis

This medicinally useful plant is also a powerful poison. The plant source of the heart drug digitalis, foxglove has been used as a natural remedy since the year 1200. A native of the Mediterranean, this plant was often used during early American times as a foundation planting around homes. It was first used as a heart medication in 1775 by the British physician attending Benjamin Franklin. It works by slowing and strengthening the heart, increasing its efficiency, while reducing congestion in the veins and inducing the kidneys to produce more urine.

As beneficial as this plant is as a drug, all of its parts—and especially the leaves—are poisonous. Even very small amounts of foxglove leaves, flowers, or other parts can dangerously disrupt the heart's rhythm. Larger amounts can stop the heart completely. Most cases of poisoning with this plant have been caused by a therapeutic drug overdose or by drinking foxglove herbal tea. Children have been poisoned by sucking on its flowers or swallowing the seeds.

SYMPTOMS OF POISONING

Within 20 to 30 minutes, a child who has ingested foxglove may experience nausea and vomiting, diarrhea, stomach pain, severe headache, blurred vision, appetite loss, irregular heartbeat, delirium, tremors, and convulsions. Death from paralysis of the heart muscle is possible, but unusual. Keep in mind, also, that anyone with very sensitive skin can develop a rash just from handling this plant.

WHAT TO DO

If you suspect your child has ingested foxglove, or even touched the plant to her mouth, call the regional Poison Control Center (1-800-222-1222) immediately. The staff at the poison center will determine if the exposure was serious enough to warrant a visit to the hospital. Do not administer anything to your child by mouth unless directed to do so by the center. If your child is not responsive (comatose) or is having seizures, call 911.

AT THE HOSPITAL

If a child who has ingested this plant is taken to the hospital within the first couple of hours, can safely swallow, and isn't continuously vomiting, the recommended initial treatment is activated charcoal. Electrolyte replacement and intravenous fluids may be necessary if dehydration develops. If there is a high blood level of potassium, abnormal heart rhythms, or low blood pressure, an antidote for digoxin (the poison in foxglove) may be administered. Atropine may be necessary to slow the heart rate.

In rare cases when the blood pressure becomes too low, drugs such as dopamine or phenylephrine may be used to raise blood pressure. In the worst cases, life support using a breathing machine may be necessary.

HEMLOCK, POISON

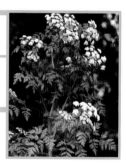

SCIENTIFIC NAME
Conium maculatum

Hemlock—which looks a lot like the carrot plant—can be rapidly fatal, as Socrates discovered in ancient Athens. The lacy leaves are the most toxic when hemlock is flowering, but all parts of this plant, also known as "fool's parsley," are poisonous. Its seeds have been mistaken for anise. Hemlock contains coniine, which acts like potent nicotine.

Quail sometimes eat hemlock seeds and pass on the poison to anyone eating the flesh of the bird. Hemlock poisoning is responsible for many human fatalities.

SYMPTOMS OF POISONING

Usually within 30 minutes after eating poison hemlock, a person will begin to develop nausea, vomiting, and abdominal pain. This can progress to weakness, muscular pain, paralysis, blindness, seizures, and breathing problems. Death typically comes within several hours as a result of respiratory paralysis.

WHAT TO DO

If you suspect your child has swallowed this plant, call the regional Poison Control Center (1-800-222-1222) immediately. The staff at the poison center will determine if the exposure was serious enough to warrant a visit to the hospital. Do not administer anything by mouth unless directed to do so by the poison center. If the child who has ingested the plant is not responsive (comatose) or is having seizures, call 911.

AT THE HOSPITAL

If the child comes for treatment within the first couple of hours, can safely swallow, and does not have continuous vomiting, the recommended initial treatment is activated charcoal. Electrolyte replacement and intravenous fluids may be necessary if dehydration occurs. If the child has lots of respiratory secretions or the heart rate becomes too slow, atropine administration may be necessary. Seizures may be treated with benzodiazepines such as diazepam. In the worst cases, life support by breathing machine may be necessary.

PLANTS

HOLLY

SCIENTIFIC NAME
Ilex

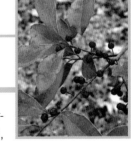

About 400 different species of the ever-popular, glossy-leafed holly, with red, white, black, yellow, or orange berries, are found in the United States. Species include Christmas holly (also called American holly) and English holly. Christmas holly is found from

Massachusetts to Florida and west to Missouri and Texas; English is cultivated from Virginia to Texas, and in the Pacific coastal states and British Columbia. Berries of all these varieties are especially poisonous, although the exact nature of the toxic chemicals is not known.

SYMPTOMS OF POISONING

In small doses, holly is a stimulant much like coffee; in larger doses, it can lead to nausea, vomiting, diarrhea, inflammation of the mouth, drowsiness, and an altered state of consciousness. The berries can be fatal to a child if eaten in large quantities.

WHAT TO DO

If you suspect your child has ingested this plant, call the regional Poison Control Center (1-800-222-1222) immediately. The staff at the poison center will determine if the exposure was serious enough to warrant a visit to the hospital. Do not administer anything by mouth unless directed to do so by the center.

AT THE HOSPITAL

If your child is taken to the hospital within the first couple of hours, can safely swallow, and isn't continually vomiting, the recommended initial treatment is activated charcoal. Electrolyte replacement and intravenous fluids may be necessary if dehydration occurs.

HYACINTH

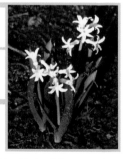

SCIENTIFIC NAME
Hyacinthus orientalis

Favored for its delicate flowers and sweet smell, this beautiful plant that comes in a variety of colors is widely grown throughout the United States. It is the hyacinth bulb that is toxic when ingested, not the flowers. Although not a deadly poison, hyacinth nonetheless can cause discomfort to a curious child whose lips even touch the bulb before it is planted in the ground.

SYMPTOMS OF POISONING

If your child gnaws on the bulb of this plant, it will cause severe stomach problems, which—while not fatal—can be quite painful.

WHAT TO DO

If you suspect your child has ingested this plant, call the regional Poison Control Center (1-800-222-1222) immediately. The staff at the poison center will determine if the exposure was serious enough to warrant a visit to the hospital. Do not administer anything by mouth unless directed to do so by the center.

AT THE HOSPITAL

If the child gets to the hospital within the first couple of hours, can safely swallow, and doesn't have continuous vomiting, the recommended initial treatment is activated charcoal. Electrolyte replacement and intravenous fluids may be necessary if dehydration occurs.

IVY

SCIENTIFIC NAME
Hedera helix

This beautiful, sprawling green plant is typically found in shady locations where it is used as a ground cover, or growing up the sides of older homes. All parts of the ivy plant—including English ivy and other common ivies—are poisonous if eaten.

PLANTS

SYMPTOMS OF POISONING

Symptoms include a burning sensation in the throat, then nausea, vomiting, stomach pain, increased salivation, and skin irritation.

WHAT TO DO

If you suspect your child has eaten this plant, call the regional Poison Control Center (1-800-222-1222) immediately; staffers will determine if the exposure was serious enough to warrant a visit to the hospital. Do not administer anything by mouth unless directed to do so by the poison center.

AT THE HOSPITAL

Electrolyte replacement and intravenous fluids may be necessary if dehydration occurs as a result of vomiting.

JACK-IN-THE-PULPIT

SCIENTIFIC NAME
Arisaema triphyllum

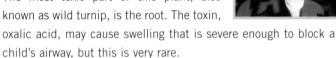

The most toxic part of this plant, also known as wild turnip, is the root. The toxin, oxalic acid, may cause swelling that is severe enough to block a child's airway, but this is very rare.

SYMPTOMS OF POISONING

Reactions after eating this plant include burning and swelling in the mouth and throat, teary eyes, and nausea and vomiting.

WHAT TO DO

If you know your child has eaten parts of this plant, wipe out his mouth with a cold, wet cloth and give him milk to drink. Wash any affected skin with water; if the eyes are involved, irrigate them with water. Call the regional Poison Control Center (1-800-222-1222) for further instructions.

AT THE HOSPITAL

Electrolyte replacement and intravenous fluids may be necessary if dehydration occurs.

JERUSALEM CHERRY

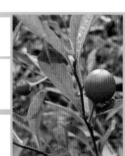

SCIENTIFIC NAME

Solanum pseudocapsicum

A member of the toxic nightshade family, this popular houseplant produces lovely but poisonous orange or red berries. Typically cultivated as a potted plant, Jerusalem cherry has escaped into the wild along the Gulf Coast and in Hawaii. Although the entire plant is poisonous, the most toxic parts are the unripened fruit and leaves. Poisoning is usually the result of eating an immature plant. While there isn't much danger of a fatal overdose in adults, young children may be at risk.

SYMPTOMS OF POISONING

Several hours after eating the berries, a child may experience stomach irritation, scratchy throat, fever, and diarrhea. Poisoning with these berries may be confused with bacterial gastroenteritis. Other symptoms include vomiting, headache, bloating, slowed breathing, central nervous system depression, confusion, and rapid heartbeat. It is unclear how many cherries would have to be eaten to cause any of these symptoms.

WHAT TO DO

If you suspect your child has swallowed this plant, call the regional Poison Control Center (1-800-222-1222) immediately; staffers will determine if the exposure was serious enough to warrant a visit to the hospital. Do not administer anything by mouth unless directed to do so by the poison center.

AT THE HOSPITAL

Electrolyte replacement and intravenous fluids may be necessary if dehydration occurs.

JESSAMINE

SCIENTIFIC NAME
Gelsemium sempervirens

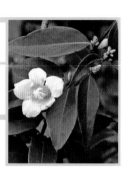

This member of the olive family includes 300 species of fragrant flowering shrubs found in woodlands in many places in North America. A perennial evergreen, jessamine has lanced leaves with fragrant bright yellow flowers. All parts of this plant—including leaves, flowers, and seeds—are toxic. There have even been cases of poisoning in children who sucked on its flowers. Honey accidentally made from the nectar of this plant has also been linked to a few fatalities.

SYMPTOMS OF POISONING

Symptoms include headache, dizziness, drooping eyelids, sweating, weakness, convulsions, anxiety, depression, and breathing failure.

WHAT TO DO

If you suspect your child has ingested this plant, call the regional Poison Control Center (1-800-222-1222) immediately; the staff will determine if the exposure was serious enough to warrant a visit to the hospital. Do not administer anything by mouth unless directed to do so by the poison center.

AT THE HOSPITAL

Activated charcoal and intravenous fluids may be required.

JIMSONWEED

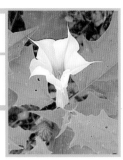

SCIENTIFIC NAME
Datura stramonium

This deadly member of the potato (or nightshade) family, which includes the poisonous plants mandrake and belladonna, is responsible for more poisonings than any other plant. It was originally called "Jamestown weed" after a mass poisoning in that Virginia town in 1666, when starving Colonial soldiers ate the seeds of the plant and became intoxicated. Also known as thorn apple, stinkweed, datura, and moonflower, this plant can poison a child who sucks the flower nectar, eats the seeds, or drinks tea made from the leaves. All parts of the jimsonweed plant are potentially toxic.

SYMPTOMS OF POISONING

Symptoms include thirst, headache, fever, dizziness, urinary retention, blurred vision, dry mouth, dilated pupils, red skin, nausea and vomiting, rapid pulse, high blood pressure, hallucinations, convulsions, and delirium.

WHAT TO DO

If you suspect your child has swallowed this plant, call the regional Poison Control Center (1-800-222-1222) immediately; the staff will determine if the exposure was serious enough to warrant a visit to the hospital. Do not administer anything by mouth unless directed to do so by the poison center.

AT THE HOSPITAL

If your child gets help within the first couple of hours, can safely swallow, and isn't continuously vomiting, the recommended initial treatment is activated charcoal. Electrolyte replacement and intravenous fluids may be necessary if dehydration occurs. A sedating benzodiazepine, such as diazepam, may be necessary to calm the patient. How sick the child becomes depends on how much was eaten, the child's age, and the time between ingestion and proper medical care. Symptoms may last for one to three days and usually require hospitalization. Death is unlikely.

JONQUIL
SEE NARCISSUS

LILY OF THE VALLEY

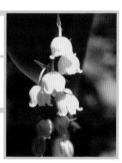

SCIENTIFIC NAME
Convallaria majalis

This lovely, shy little plant with delicate white flowers grows in damp and shady spots, but it carries a potent poison in its fruit, leaves, flowers, and roots. Even the water in which cut flowers from this plant are kept can be toxic. Although all parts of the lily of the valley are poisonous, the leaves are especially so.

The plant, which is similar to foxglove, is a hardy perennial with bell-shaped flowers hanging off its stems. It spreads by underground runners. Lily of the valley grows wild throughout North America, and may sometimes bear orange or red berries.

SYMPTOMS OF POISONING
Shortly after ingestion, the child may experience a rash, weakness, headache, nausea, and visual changes (including seeing yellow halos around objects). If larger amounts are eaten, dizziness and vomiting may occur within one or two hours. Coma and

death may result from heart failure. If the patient survives for the first 24 hours, recovery is expected.

WHAT TO DO

If you suspect your child has eaten this plant, call the regional Poison Control Center (1-800-222-1222) immediately; the staff will determine if the exposure was serious enough to warrant a visit to the hospital. Do not administer anything by mouth unless directed to do so by the poison center.

AT THE HOSPITAL

Doctors will administer activated charcoal, while monitoring vital signs and electrocardiograms. Correction of electrolyte imbalance may be required. Drugs to control heart rhythm also may be required. A specific antidote is rarely needed, but in severe cases of toxicity, it may be required.

MISTLETOE

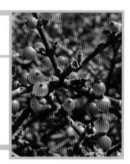

SCIENTIFIC NAMES
Phoradendron rubrum
P. serotinum
P. tomentosum

Mistletoe, a popular Christmas decorative plant, is toxic when ingested. Its stem, leaves, and white or pink berries are poisonous. *P. serotinum* is the variety usually sold as a holiday plant; it grows from New Jersey to Florida and west to southern Illinois and Texas. *P. tomentosum* grows from Kansas to Louisiana and west to Texas and Mexico.

A plant steeped in legend, it is said that the mistletoe, when a tree, provided the wood used to make Christ's cross. As a result, it was relegated to existence as a parasite, living off of other plants.

PLANTS

Its reputation as an herb of love originated in Scandinavia. According to Nordic legend, the god Balder—the god of peace—had been killed with an arrow dipped in mistletoe. When he was restored to life at the request of other gods, mistletoe was given to his mother—the goddess of love—who announced that anyone who passed under it must be given a kiss. It became part of Christmas celebrations after the Druids used the greens to welcome the New Year.

SYMPTOMS OF POISONING

Mistletoe's poison primarily affects the gastrointestinal tract. It can result in nausea, vomiting, diarrhea, and dehydration.

WHAT TO DO

If you suspect your child has ingested mistletoe, call the regional Poison Control Center (1-800-222-1222) immediately. The staff at the poison center will determine if the exposure was serious enough to warrant a visit to the hospital.

AT THE HOSPITAL

If a child who has swallowed this plant gets help within the first couple of hours, can safely swallow, and is not vomiting continuously, the recommended initial treatment is activated charcoal. Electrolyte replacement and intravenous fluids may be necessary if dehydration occurs.

MONKSHOOD

SCIENTIFIC NAME
Aconitum

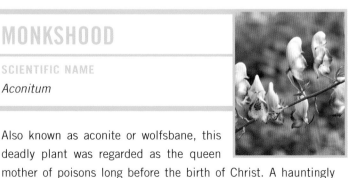

Also known as aconite or wolfsbane, this deadly plant was regarded as the queen mother of poisons long before the birth of Christ. A hauntingly beautiful garden perennial, it bears small blue, pink, or white flowers from June to September. Monkshood stands more than six feet tall, and towers over other flowers. A member of the buttercup family, it looks like a delphinium.

In the past, monkshood was used medicinally, and with the increasing popularity of herbs in the United States, *Aconitum* products now are sold in some herbal stores. The entire plant is poisonous, although the roots and leaves are the most toxic. One teaspoonful of the pure root (3–6 milligrams) can kill an adult. Because the root looks very much like horseradish or a Jerusalem artichoke, monkshood should never be planted in a vegetable garden.

SYMPTOMS OF POISONING

As soon as monkshood is eaten, a burning or tingling sensation begins in the lips, tongue, mouth, fingers, and toes. This gradually spreads throughout the entire body, but is reportedly particularly strong in the facial area. These symptoms are followed by temporary excessive salivation, then a dry mouth, accompanied by nausea, vomiting, a sensation of throat constriction, difficulty in swallowing, or speech problems. Pupils may dilate, and there may be temporary visual disturbances including blurry vision or color distortion. Dizziness, prickling skin, and muscle weakness may occur.

In severe poisoning, there may be disturbances in heart rate and rhythm, followed by convulsions and death. Death may occur as quickly as a few minutes after ingestion of the plant or several days later.

WHAT TO DO

If you suspect monkshood poisoning, call the regional Poison Control Center number (1-800-222-1222) immediately. The staff at the poison center will determine if the exposure was serious enough to warrant a visit to the hospital.

AT THE HOSPITAL

Electrolyte replacement and intravenous fluids may be necessary if dehydration occurs. Medications to halt seizures and to reverse heart disturbances may be administered. Life support may be necessary in the worst poisonings.

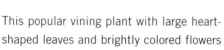

MORNING GLORY

SCIENTIFIC NAME
Ipomoea

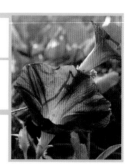

This popular vining plant with large heart-shaped leaves and brightly colored flowers was cultivated in the past for its hallucinogenic properties. In particular, the Aztecs and various North American Indians used the morning glory as part of their religious ceremonies, for healing, and in divination. In more recent times, the seeds have been used as a hallucinogen. The seeds, which are poisonous, contain an active ingredient similar to the illegal street drug lysergic acid diethylamide (LSD).

SYMPTOMS OF POISONING

Only mildly toxic if eaten, this plant primarily causes hallucinations, along with dilated pupils, nausea and vomiting, diarrhea, drowsiness, numbness, and muscle tightness. However, between 50 and 200 powdered seeds must be eaten to produce symptoms. Flashbacks may occur later.

WHAT TO DO

If you suspect an overdose, call the regional Poison Control Center (1-800-222-1222) immediately. The staff at the poison center will determine if the exposure was serious enough to warrant a visit to the hospital.

AT THE HOSPITAL

Electrolyte replacement and intravenous fluids may be necessary if dehydration occurs as a result of vomiting.

MOTHER-IN-LAW PLANT

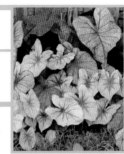

SCIENTIFIC NAME
Caladium

This popular indoor and outdoor plant has arrow-shaped leaves that come in a range of colors from white to green or red. It belongs to a group of plants that contain oxylates. All parts of this plant are toxic, and can irritate the mouth if eaten.

SYMPTOMS OF POISONING

Eating this plant causes irritation and swelling of the mouth, lips, throat, and digestive tract, which can lead to nausea, vomiting, or diarrhea. Eating a very large amount can cause more serious swelling that may obstruct the airway.

WHAT TO DO

Call the regional Poison Control Center (1-800-222-1222) immediately; the staff will determine if the exposure was serious enough to warrant a visit to the hospital. Give the child cool liquids (such as milk) to hold in the mouth to ease the pain. Painkillers may be given, but eventually the pain and swelling subside on their own. If your child feels as if the airway is swelling or has trouble breathing, call 911.

AT THE HOSPITAL

Electrolyte replacement and intravenous fluids may be necessary if dehydration occurs.

NARCISSUS

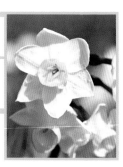

SCIENTIFIC NAME
Narcissus

This familiar yellow flower, also known as daffodil (*N. pseudonarcissus)* or jonquil (*N. jonquilla*), includes about 26 varieties and hundreds of cultivars. It's often planted in masses in lawns and gardens throughout the United States. According to ancient Greek mythology, this is the plant that grew on the spot where the handsome Narcissus saw his own reflection, became so enamored of it that he couldn't leave the spot, and died there. The beautiful flower—the "flower of death"—is said to have grown from the spot where his head dropped.

Narcissus is a welcome harbinger of spring in many locations, but most homeowners are totally unaware that these beautiful plants are also toxic. Even the water in a vase in which the flowers are kept may be toxic. While native to central Europe and North Africa, these plants are grown everywhere in the United States.

The most poisonous part of the plant is the bulb, which contains the toxin lycorine. If eaten, it can cause vomiting, diarrhea, and convulsions. If eaten in large amounts, it could cause death in humans and animals.

PREVENTION!

Bulbs should be planted right away. Wear garden gloves when planting, as handling the bulb can cause skin irritation in sensitive people.

SYMPTOMS OF POISONING

Just eating a small part of this plant or its bulb can cause poisoning, even in an adult. Within a few hours after ingestion, your child may experience nausea, vomiting, diarrhea, and abdominal pain. A skin irritation may occur in sensitive individuals who handle the bulbs, flowers, and stems.

WHAT TO DO

If you suspect your child has eaten this plant (especially the bulb), call the regional Poison Control Center (1-800-222-1222) immediately. The staff at the poison center will determine if the exposure was serious enough to warrant a visit to the hospital.

AT THE HOSPITAL

Electrolyte replacement and intravenous fluids may be necessary if dehydration occurs as a result of vomiting.

PLANTS

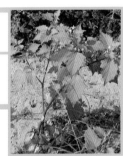

NIGHTSHADE, BLACK

SCIENTIFIC NAME
Solanum nigrum

A member of the Solanaceae family (which includes many toxic members), this true nightshade contains the poison solanine. Its cousin, deadly nightshade (see: Nightshade, deadly), contains the poison atropine. Because solanine and atropine have different effects on the body, reporting an incident as "nightshade poisoning" isn't specific enough to determine an exact course of treatment. Solanine is potentially toxic even in small quantities, and the toxin is found throughout the plant—especially in the unripened fruit and leaves.

SYMPTOMS OF POISONING

The most common effects are nausea, vomiting, headache, and diarrhea. Drowsiness, delirium, and coma may occur, but are exceedingly rare.

WHAT TO DO

If you suspect your child has eaten this plant, call the regional Poison Control Center number (1-800-222-1222) immediately; the staff will determine if the exposure was serious enough to warrant a visit to the hospital.

AT THE HOSPITAL

If a child who has swallowed this plant gets help within the first couple of hours, can safely swallow, and doesn't have continuous vomiting, the recommended initial treatment is activated charcoal. Electrolyte replacement and intravenous fluids may be necessary if dehydration occurs.

NIGHTSHADE, DEADLY

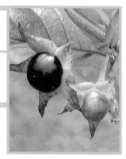

SCIENTIFIC NAME
Atropa belladonna

Also known as belladonna, this powerfully toxic plant has a history rich in legend and magic. A member of the Solanaceae family (which includes many toxic members), deadly nightshade contains the poison atropine. Its cousins, the true nightshades (see: Jerusalem cherry and Nightshade, black), contain the poison solanine. Because solanine and atropine have different effects on the body, reporting an incident as "nightshade poisoning" isn't specific enough to determine how to treat the patient.

Found throughout North America in shady, marshy places, the deadly nightshade is cultivated commercially in Europe for its medicinal properties. Its glossy black berries and bell-shaped flowers give off a sweet smell from July through September. The entire plant is toxic, but ingesting a single berry can be deadly. The root is the most poisonous part of the entire plant, containing a higher percentage of toxic tropane alkaloids. However, the berries are the biggest risk to a child, because they are sweet. A child is much more likely to eat a berry than chomp the root.

SYMPTOMS OF POISONING

Symptoms usually appear within an hour after eating and include a scratching or burning feeling in the throat, rapid pulse, fever, nausea, vomiting, blurred vision, dilated pupils, inability to urinate, problems swallowing, mental confusion, hallucinations, aggressive behavior, convulsions, coma, and death.

WHAT TO DO

If you suspect your child has eaten this plant, call the regional Poison Control Center (1-800-222-1222) immediately; the staff will determine if the exposure was serious enough to warrant a visit to the hospital.

AT THE HOSPITAL

If the victim gets help within the first couple of hours, can safely swallow, and does not have continuous vomiting, the recommended initial treatment is activated charcoal. Electrolyte replacement and intravenous fluids may be necessary if dehydration occurs. Life support may be necessary in the worst cases.

OLEANDER, WHITE AND YELLOW

SCIENTIFIC NAMES
Nerium oleander
Thevetia peruviana

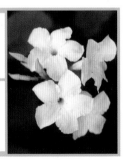

Widely cultivated in the United States as fragrant ornamental shrubs and houseplants, both types of oleander are deadly. White oleander has white, yellow, pink, or red blossoms; yellow oleander's blossoms are yellow with a hint of peach.

PLANTS

All parts of the plant are poisonous. The nectar from the flowers, honey from the pollen, smoke from the burning plants, and water in which the cut flowers are kept are also potentially toxic. Cases of poisoning have been reported from eating hot dogs roasted over a fire on oleander twigs.

SYMPTOMS OF POISONING

Symptoms may begin immediately after swallowing any part of this plant, and include nausea, vomiting, abdominal pain, diarrhea, dizziness, slow or irregular heartbeat, and dilated pupils. This may be followed by slowed breathing, coma, and death.

WHAT TO DO

If you suspect your child has eaten this plant, call the regional Poison Control Center (1-800-222-1222) immediately; the staff will determine if the exposure was serious enough to warrant a visit to the hospital.

AT THE HOSPITAL

If the victim gets to the hospital within the first couple of hours, can safely swallow, and does not have continuous vomiting, the recommended initial treatment is activated charcoal. Electrolyte replacement and intravenous fluids may be necessary if dehydration occurs. An antidote may be given if the victim develops significant heart symptoms or a high potassium level.

PHILODENDRON

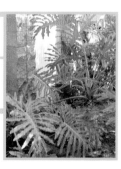

SCIENTIFIC NAME
Monstera deliciosa

One of the most common houseplants, philodendron is widely favored for its indestructible nature and attractive, glossy green leaves. But the plant contains oxylates that cause marked irritation if eaten.

SYMPTOMS OF POISONING

Immediately after eating the leaves, the child's mouth, lips, and throat will burn and swell. Because pain is triggered so quickly, there is little risk that a child will consume large amounts.

WHAT TO DO

Call the regional Poison Control Center (1-800-222-1222) immediately and the staff will tell you what to do. Poisoning from this plant rarely requires more than home care. Typically, the pain and swelling will subside without treatment. Cool liquids (such as milk) or a cold, wet cloth held in the mouth can ease the pain.

POISON IVY, POISON OAK, AND POISON SUMAC

SCIENTIFIC NAME
Toxicodendron radicans

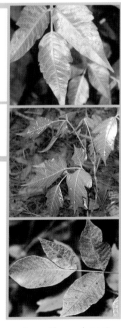

These are some of the most familiar and widespread plants in the United States, and they are all toxic. Found in woodsy areas throughout the country, the common poison ivy (top), poison oak (middle), and poison sumac (bottom) irritate the skin of most people who touch them.

Fortunately, the most common—poison ivy—has glossy green leaves that are fairly easy to notice, almost

PLANTS

always growing in groups of three ("leaves of three, let them be") two leaves opposite each other, and one at the end of the stalk.

Poison ivy, oak, and sumac are closely related plants that all contain the colorless resin urushiol. While each plant contains a slightly different form of urushiol, they are so similar that children sensitive to one will react to all three. The entire plant contains this resin—leaves, berries, stalks, and roots. It's easy to transfer urushiol from one object to another or to another person, which means that anything that touches these plants—whether the hands, gardening gloves or tools, a pet's fur, a sleeping bag—can be contaminated and cause a reaction. Moreover, urushiol remains active for at least a year. Even the smoke from burning these plants is toxic and can irritate the skin, eyes, or lungs. The leaves also can irritate the throat if eaten.

As the leaves die in the fall, the oil still remains active—this means that even during the winter you can be affected by the urushiol if you use wood containing stems from any of these twining plants.

Touching any of these three actually triggers an allergic reaction to the plant's sap (urushiol). About seven out of 10 people are sensitive to the sap, and will develop a contact skin irritation. Children often do not react to their first contact with these plants, but most will develop the allergy upon subsequent exposure.

PREVENTION!

There are effective commercial products that can help keep urushiol oil from getting into the skin. Alternatively, you could try what seems to work for some U.S. Forestry Service employees—spray some deodorant on your arms and legs before venturing out into an area rife with these plants. According to some dermatologists, the active ingredient in antiperspirant deodorants (aluminum chlorohydrate) can prevent urushiol from irritating the skin.

POISON IVY MYTHS

Despite common misconceptions, poison ivy is not spread by scratching open blisters or by touching the irritated skin of a person who has a poison ivy rash—as long as no oil is present. Only the urushiol sap itself can trigger a reaction.

Typically, the rash does not appear all at once, but may worsen over the course of several days, which leads to the misconception that the rash is "spreading" by touch. Only if the urushiol has not been washed off could touching the blisters spread the rash to another part of the body.

SYMPTOMS OF POISONING

Skin reactions may vary in different children; some individuals experience a mild itching, while others suffer from severe burning and itching with many large, watery blisters. The skin irritation and blistering may appear within hours or days after touching the plants, but usually develop within 24 to 48 hours in those who are sensitive. Typically, the rash peaks within five days, and gradually improves over a week or two, even without treatment. Eventually the blisters break and the oozing sores crust over and then disappear.

In some cases, allergy to poison ivy, oak, or sumac may mean a child is also allergic to the fruits of related plants, including cashews, pistachios, and mangos.

WHAT TO DO

As soon as possible after your child touches one of these plants, you should wash the affected area (within 10 minutes if possible) with soap and water. Do not bathe your child in a tub, as this could spread the oil, and don't scrub the affected area with a brush. If the urushiol is washed off in time, further treatment isn't usually necessary.

If contaminated while in an isolated area outdoors, wash the affected skin in a cold running stream. Any clothing that may have come in contact with the plants or the oil must be washed several times.

Once itching develops, apply cold compresses. It is the fastest and cheapest way to temporarily soothe the discomfort. Put calamine lotion on the rash to help ease the itching and burning, and dry the skin.

AT THE HOSPITAL

In cases of severe skin reaction, or if the rash is all over the child's body, face, or in the genital area, your child should be seen by a doctor, who may prescribe antihistamines and topical or oral steroids. All of these can effectively treat the rash and itching. Injected corticosteroids are most helpful when they are given quickly after the rash appears; topical corticosteroids aren't recommended for weeping or blistered rashes.

RHUBARB

SCIENTIFIC NAME
Rheum rhabarbarum

Although the reddish stalk of this plant is a popular food enjoyed in a variety of cooked or stewed ways, the leaves are toxic. They must be removed before cooking or eating rhubarb.

SYMPTOMS OF POISONING

Several hours after ingestion, the irritant in the leaves can cause a burning sensation in the mouth, abdominal pain, nausea, vomiting, and breathing difficulty. In rare cases, people who have eaten the leaves have developed bloody urine, back pain, and kidney problems, all of which can be cured with proper medical care.

WHAT TO DO

If your child has eaten the leaves of a rhubarb plant, call the regional Poison Control Center (1-800-222-1222) immediately; the staff will determine if the exposure was serious enough to warrant a visit to the hospital.

AT THE HOSPITAL

Electrolyte replacement and intravenous fluids may be necessary if dehydration occurs as a result of vomiting.

TOMATO PLANT

SCIENTIFIC NAME
Lycopersicon esculentum

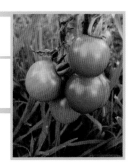

Although the fruit of the tomato plant is a tasty and highly prized summer vegetable, the leaves and roots can be poisonous if eaten. The tomato is a member of the nightshade class of plants, meaning it contains the toxin solanine. Other plants within this group include the potato, black nightshade, and eggplant.

SYMPTOMS OF POISONING

If ingested, this plant can cause headache, nausea, vomiting, diarrhea, and, occasionally, drowsiness.

PLANTS

If you suspect your child has eaten the leaves or root of this plant, call the regional Poison Control Center (1-800-222-1222). The staff will determine if the exposure was serious enough to warrant a visit to the hospital.

AT THE HOSPITAL
Electrolyte replacement and intravenous fluids may be necessary if dehydration occurs as a result of vomiting.

YEW

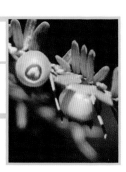

SCIENTIFIC NAME
Taxus

Several types of yew tree are poisonous, including the English yew (*T. baccata*), the Pacific or western yew (*T. brevifolia*), the American yew or ground hemlock (*T. canadensis*), and the Japanese yew (*T. cuspidata*). In ancient times, parts of the yew tree were used to induce abortions, with often tragic results.

Found throughout the northern hemisphere, all parts of this evergreen shrub are poisonous, except for the red berries. Although the berries aren't poisonous, the seeds inside them are potentially toxic. However, the human digestive system is unable to break down the seeds, so if they are swallowed whole, no poison will be released and they will be eliminated from the body.

SYMPTOMS OF POISONING
Symptoms will appear about an hour after ingestion and include dizziness, dry mouth, nausea, vomiting, diarrhea, and abdominal pain. This may be followed by breathing problems, muscle weakness, slow heartbeat, convulsions, shock, or coma. It may ultimately lead to respiratory failure and death.

WHAT TO DO

If you suspect your child has eaten any part of this plant, call the regional Poison Control Center (1-800-222-1222) immediately; the staff will determine if the exposure was serious enough to warrant a visit to the hospital.

AT THE HOSPITAL

If the child gets help within the first couple of hours, can safely swallow, and does not have continuous vomiting, the recommended initial treatment is activated charcoal. Electrolyte replacement and intravenous fluids may be necessary if dehydration occurs. Life support may be necessary in the worst cases.

POISONOUS MUSHROOMS

There are more than 5,000 varieties of mushrooms found in the United States, but only about 100 types of these fleshy fungi are toxic. Most of the severe poisonings are caused by eating the wrong type of mushrooms that people have picked in the woods. Most calls to poison centers are from parents whose children have eaten a mushroom in the wild, but these rarely cause symptoms. If they do, it's usually only an upset stomach. Often it's impossible to identify by appearance the type of mushroom that was eaten, but because toxic mushrooms only produce a few distinct syndromes, an expert, known as a mycologist, can usually identify the type of mushroom by the kind of symptoms the person is experiencing.

A few types of mushrooms are considered deadly, and eating these can be fatal. Most poison mushrooms, however, cause gastrointestinal irritation that triggers typical nausea, vomiting, and diarrhea. These symptoms usually appear quickly. If symptoms appear within two hours of eating mushrooms, they are rarely severe and don't usually require hospital treatment. But if symptoms develop more than six hours later, experts normally suspect a more serious poisoning involving amatoxin or monomethylhydrazine.

The science of mycology, unfortunately, is not exact. Since the first report of mushroom poisoning in 1871, most of the "rules" about detecting toxic mushrooms have been proven inaccurate. In fact, there is no rule that applies to all species of mushrooms. For example, it's not true that if you place a silver coin or silver spoon in a pan of mushrooms on the stove, the silver will turn black if the mushrooms are poisonous. Any rotten mushroom in boiling water will discolor silver, but no fresh mushroom will do so, whether it's poisonous or not. Moreover, poisonous mushrooms won't look milky if you soak them in vinegar, and they won't get darker if you soak them in water.

Only an experienced mycologist can truly tell the difference between a safe and a poisonous mushroom, because the toxicity of mushrooms is quite complex. Some are always potentially deadly; others are poisonous only at certain times in their growth stage. Some mushrooms have never been regarded as toxic simply because no one has ever eaten them.

WHAT TO TELL THE DOCTOR

If you suspect that someone in your family has eaten a poisonous mushroom, get the details so you will be prepared to answer these questions that the doctor or poison center expert will ask:

> ✕ When was the mushroom eaten, and when did symptoms appear?

> ✕ What are the symptoms and which appeared first? Are symptoms mostly nausea and vomiting? Is there stomach pain?

> ✕ Is the person experiencing hallucinations?

> ✕ Is the person sweating?

> ✕ Is the person able to urinate?

IT MAY JUST BE AN ALLERGY!

Some people are simply allergic to mushrooms. Others have inherited an inability to handle the unusual sugars found in mushrooms. Both can cause gas and diarrhea.

COPRINE CLASS

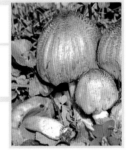

SCIENTIFIC NAME
Coprinus

The toxin in this class of mushrooms is coprine, which blocks a liver enzyme called acetaldehyde dehydrogenase. Coprine is found in the *Coprinus atramentarius* mushroom (also known as inky caps) and a few other more rare species of the same genus.

SYMPTOMS OF POISONING
Eating this mushroom won't cause any symptoms unless the person also drinks alcohol within several days of eating the mushroom. If coprine is in the system, even a small amount of alcohol can cause acetaldehyde to build up in the blood. Symptoms appear between 30 minutes and two hours after drinking alcohol, and include flushing, rapid heart rate, low blood pressure, nausea, and vomiting. Death is rare.

WHAT TO DO
Contact the regional Poison Control Center (1-800-222-1222) immediately. The staff at the center will determine if the exposure was serious enough to warrant a visit to the hospital.

Treatment involves reducing the symptoms and may require replacement of fluids and electrolytes.

CYCLOPEPTIDE CLASS

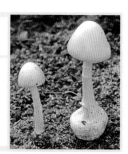

SCIENTIFIC NAMES
Amanita phalloides
Amanita verna
Amanita virosa

The most common poisonous mushrooms in the United States are those in the genus *Amanita*. Some of these are among the most deadly in the world, and include the death angel (*Amanita verna*); destroying angel (*Amanita virosa*), pictured above; and—most deadly of all—the death cap (*Amanita phalloides*). The poisonous substance is a toxin called cyclopeptide. Even though the exact percentage is not known, many people throughout the world die each year as a result of eating mushrooms in this class. Between 25 and 35 types of *Amanitas* are found in the United States. However, experts disagree about the exact classification of many of the *Amanita* mushrooms, because they are so closely related.

The *Amanitas* usually have white spores, a ringed stem, a veil, and a cup from which the stalk grows. Those that are snow white to pale green or tan are particularly dangerous.

Mushrooms in this group contain a number of different cyclopeptides within two primary groups: amatoxins and phallotoxins. A mortality rate of between 10 and 60 percent has been reported, but this may be skewed by the fact that milder cases—involving only nausea and diarrhea—probably go unreported.

SYMPTOMS OF POISONING
Symptoms usually appear six to 10 hours after ingestion and

include sudden nausea, vomiting, and severe diarrhea that may contain blood and mucus. The diarrhea may be so severe that the symptoms appear very much like cholera. Other symptoms may include dehydration and jaundice, a yellowing of the skin. The victim may then appear to recover, but two to four days later may experience liver, heart, and kidney damage. Circulatory failure, convulsions, coma, and death may follow.

WHAT TO DO

Contact the regional Poison Control Center (1-800-222-1222) immediately. The staff at the center will determine if the exposure was serious enough to warrant a visit to the hospital.

AT THE HOSPITAL

People who have ingested these mushrooms may be given activated charcoal. N-acetylcysteine may be given if liver toxicity develops. Silibinin, which is derived from milk thistle, has been used to treat this type of mushroom poisoning in Europe, though it is not currently available in the United States. In addition, a high dose of penicillin may be given to block the toxin. In cases of severe kidney failure, dialysis may be recommended.

GASTROINTESTINAL IRRITANT CLASS

SCIENTIFIC NAME
Chlorophyllum molybdites

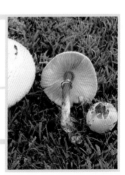

You may well find this beautiful poisonous mushroom popping up in clusters on your front lawn in the summer or fall. The gills of mature specimens have a distinctive green color. Poisoning from the *Chlorophyllum molybdite,* commonly called a green gill, is quite common in North America, because the mushroom is so large, attractive, and available.

Experienced mushroom hunters have often mistaken it for closely related edible mushrooms such as *C. rhacodes* or *Macrolepiota procera.*

SYMPTOMS OF POISONING

Symptoms typically begin within the first few hours after eating, and include nausea and vomiting. Diarrhea also may occur. Death is rare, and fatal cases are usually due to dehydration and electrolyte imbalances caused by diarrhea and vomiting, especially in sick, very young, or very old patients.

WHAT TO DO

Contact the regional Poison Control Center (1-800-222-1222) immediately. The staff at the center will determine if the exposure was serious enough to warrant a visit to the hospital.

AT THE HOSPITAL

Treatment includes monitoring and treating symptoms.

HALLUCINOGENIC CLASS

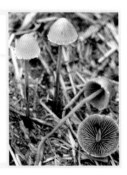

SCIENTIFIC NAMES

Conocybe
Panaeolus
Psilocybe
Stropharia

Hallucinogenic mushrooms are important to the sacred ceremonies of the American Indians, but they are also favored by drug abusers for the hallucinations they produce. The toxin in this class of mushrooms is psilocybin, which affects the central nervous system.

These mushrooms include four main groups: the *psilocybes* (*P. caeruylescens, P. mexicana, P. pelliculosa, P. cyanescens, P. baeo-*

cystis, P. cubensis); the *conocybes* (*C. cyanopus, C. smithii*); the *stropharias* (*S. cubensis*); and the *panaeolus* (*P. subbalteatus*). All produce visual and auditory hallucinations.

SYMPTOMS OF POISONING

Symptoms begin between 15 minutes and one hour after eating, and include enlarged pupils, drowsiness, concentration problems, dizziness, muscle weakness, difficulty walking, and hallucinations. Death is rare.

The hallucinogenic effects depend on how much of the mushroom is eaten, and may vary from one person to the next. Both space and time distortions have been reported, together with visual and auditory hallucinations. The period of intoxication is not usually very long (typically between three and six hours). However, there is a danger that the person may become destructive during the hallucinogenic experience.

WHAT TO DO

Contact the regional Poison Control Center (1-800-222-1222) immediately. The staff at the center will determine if the exposure was serious enough to warrant a visit to the hospital.

AT THE HOSPITAL

Treatment includes monitoring and treating the symptoms. Benzodiazepines such as Valium may be needed for sedation.

MONOMETHYLHYDRAZINE CLASS

SCIENTIFIC NAME
Gyromitra esculenta

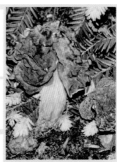

Many varieties of the *Gyromitra* mushroom (also known as the false morel) contain gyromitrin, which after being absorbed in the body is broken down to monomethylhydrazine, a toxin that affects the central nervous system. (It's also used as a component in rocket fuel.)

Even though the toxin dissolves readily in water, these mushrooms should not be eaten. This species has no gills, and its spores develop in tiny sacs on the surfaces of the fruiting bodies. It gets its nickname ("brain fungus") from its appearance, and while many species of *Gyromitra* are edible, only an expert can tell the difference.

The reported poisoning mortality rate ranges between 15 and 40 percent. However, this may be inflated by the fact that people with mild symptoms probably don't report the incident.

SYMPTOMS OF POISONING

Symptoms appear between six and 10 hours after ingestion; they include weakness, abdominal pain, nausea, and vomiting, and can lead to seizures, kidney and liver failure, and methemoglobinemia (a blood disorder).

WHAT TO DO

Contact the regional Poison Control Center (1-800-222-1222) immediately. The staff at the center will determine if the exposure was serious enough to warrant a visit to the hospital.

AT THE HOSPITAL

Poisoning involving this type of mushroom is treated with intravenous pyridoxine (vitamin B6) and benzodiazepines, such as Valium.

MUSCARINE CLASS

SCIENTIFIC NAMES

Boletus
Clitocybe
Inocybe

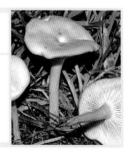

The toxin in this class of mushrooms is muscarine, which affects the autonomic nervous system, the part that regulates involuntary functions of the body. Cooking will not kill the mushroom's toxicity. The mushrooms known to contain the highest content of these toxins include *Boletus, Clitocybe,* and *Inocybe.* These mushrooms are characterized by gray-brown spores and small brown caps, and they can be found in pine forests throughout the United States.

SYMPTOMS OF POISONING

Symptoms begin between 30 minutes and two hours after ingestion and include sweating, wheezing, small pupils, increased salivation, tearing, and involuntary urination and defecation. Death from eating these types of mushrooms is rare.

WHAT TO DO

Contact the regional Poison Control Center (1-800-222-1222) immediately. The staff at the center will determine if the exposure was serious enough to warrant a visit to the hospital.

AT THE HOSPITAL

Treatment consists of intravenous atropine, a drug used to counteract the toxin.

MUSCIMOL/ IBOTENIC ACID CLASS

SCIENTIFIC NAMES
Amanita muscaria
Amanita pantherina

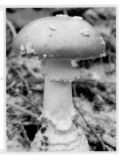

The toxins in this type of mushroom are ibotenic acid and muscimol, which affect the central nervous system. *Amanita muscaria* is also known as fly agaric because it attracts flies, which die when they come in contact with the mushroom. These mushrooms were ingested for thousands of years for their hallucinogenic properties.

SYMPTOMS OF POISONING

Symptoms begin between 30 minutes and two hours after eating, and include dizziness, impaired coordination, hallucinations, delirium, and seizures. Death from eating this kind of mushroom is rare.

WHAT TO DO

Contact the regional Poison Control Center (1-800-222-1222) immediately. The staff at the center will determine if the exposure was serious enough to warrant a visit to the hospital.

AT THE HOSPITAL

Benzodiazepines (such as Valium) may be given for sedation or to treat seizures.

ORELLINE CLASS

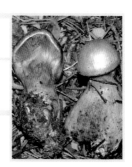

SCIENTIFIC NAME

Cortinarius

These mushrooms can be as deadly as the toxic *Amanita* class; a little more than a cup of the cooked mushrooms can be fatal. The caps range in color from bluish violet to brown or red. The toxins in this class of mushrooms are orelline and orellanin, which primarily affect the kidneys, although the liver also may be affected.

SYMPTOMS OF POISONING

Symptoms do not begin until at least 24 hours after eating, and may not start until three days to two weeks after ingestion. By then, the person usually has developed a fierce thirst, and may be drinking several quarts of fluid a day. At this point, the liver and kidneys may be irreversibly damaged. Symptoms include nausea and vomiting, headache, muscular aches, chills, decreased urine formation, and kidney failure.

WHAT TO DO

Contact the regional Poison Control Center (1-800-222-1222) immediately. The staff at the center will determine if the exposure was serious enough to warrant a visit to the hospital.

AT THE HOSPITAL

Treatment includes monitoring and treating the symptoms. The quicker the symptoms are treated, the better the outlook for survival.

MUSHROOMS

4

STEER CLEAR

POISONOUS SNAKES AND TOADS

Snakes rarely evoke a lukewarm response from humans. We may find them sinuously beautiful and yet, almost by instinct, we are repelled by them. Despite our inborn fears, most snakes are harmless, and play important roles in the fragile ecosystems of the nation's wild areas. Nevertheless, every state but Maine, Alaska, and Hawaii harbors at least one type of poisonous snake. So if your family hikes, camps, or picnics in snake-inhabited areas, you should never forget the potential danger. A bite from one of the four varieties of poisonous snakes found in the United States should always be treated as a medical emergency.

While snakebites are not uncommon in the United States—about 8,000 Americans are treated for snakebite each year—only about five people are killed by them annually. The highest reported death rates are in Arizona, Florida, Georgia, Texas, and Alabama.

There are just two families of venomous snakes native to the United States: the *Crotalidae* and the *Elapidae*. The vast majority are pit vipers in the family *Crotalidae*—a group that includes rattlesnakes, copperheads, and water moccasins. (For a detailed discussion of water moccasins, see page 193). Pit vipers get their common name from a small heat-detecting "pit" between the eye and nostril that allows the snake to sense prey at night. Almost all of the venomous bites in this country are inflicted by pit vipers. Some of these snakes, such as the Mojave or canebrake rattlesnakes, inject neurotoxin venom that attacks the muscles. Copperheads have milder and less dangerous venom that is seldom fatal in adults but can be very dangerous in children.

The seriousness of a bite depends on the snake's size (usually the larger, the more poisonous), the angle, depth, and length of the bite, and its location on the body. Bites on the head and trunk are more serious than those on limbs, and bites on the arms are more serious than those on the legs. The size and health of the victim also affects the outcome; children, infants, and the elderly are at higher risk, as are people with diabetes, high blood pressure, or blood coagulation problems.

The amount of venom delivered by a pit viper bite varies. These snakes have a very sophisticated mechanism designed to deliver venom at the exact instant its teeth are sunk into the flesh. If the snake's timing is off, however, venom is released prematurely. About 30 percent of the time, humans escape a venomous bite because of an uncoordinated attack.

There are two species of coral snakes, which are found primarily in the south. The coral snake's small mouth and short teeth make its venom delivery much less efficient than pit vipers. In fact, if your child is bitten by a coral snake, you might not even be able to see any fang marks, which can make the bite hard to detect. Coral snakebites are rare in the United States (an average of only about 25 a year), but the venom they inject can be highly toxic.

Any snakebite warrants medical attention, especially since some nonpoisonous snakes (such as the scarlet king snake) mimic the coloring of poisonous varieties. Because many people who are bitten can't positively identify the type of snake, you should seek prompt care for any bite, even if you think the snake is nonpoisonous. Keep in mind, too, that even a bite from a so-called harmless snake can cause an infection or allergic reaction in some individuals.

Fortunately, the bites of both pit vipers and coral snakes can be effectively treated with antivenin, as long as you get to the hospital quickly—within 30 minutes is best.

FIRST AID FOR SNAKEBITE

Snakebite first aid is rife with myths and dangerous bits of advice. The most important actions to take for a snakebite victim are to immobilize the bitten area and quickly transport the person for evaluation by trained medical personnel.

Many first aid measures for snakebite that were taught in the past are no longer recommended. Likewise, it's no longer recommended that bystanders try to capture the snake for identification—that may only lead to yet another victim. In any case, no matter what species was involved, a doctor's thorough examination and proper observation of the victim will dictate treatment. The bystander's focus always should be directed toward getting professional medical care as quickly as possible, not snaring the snake or trying to treat the victim at the scene.

 You should avoid making incisions through the wound, applying suction devices or tourniquets, employing electric shock therapy, or applying cold or warm compresses. Ice or ice water should not be applied directly to the wound; this is of no proven value and actually may cause more injury.

WHAT TO DO

In addition to seeking help immediately, you should remove any jewelry near the bite site because swelling might make it difficult to remove later. Reassure the person and try to keep him calm and still, since increased physical activity may hasten the spread of venom.

AT THE HOSPITAL

As soon as possible, trained professionals should evaluate the snakebite victim to assess whether antivenin is needed. Other treatments may include a tetanus shot, some form of transfusion, intravenous fluids, and antiemetics (medications to prevent vomiting) to counteract the nausea caused by many snakebites. Antibiotics are rarely given, because snakebite wounds are unlikely to become infected.

RATTLESNAKES

Rattlesnakes come in different sizes and colors, and all resemble other vipers in their family, with one important difference—the telltale rattle at the end of their tails. The rattle is formed by a series of dry segments that the snake uses to warn of its presence.

Although rattlesnakes are poisonous, fatalities are rare, because antivenin is usually readily available at hospitals. While most rattlers are concentrated in the southwestern United States, they are also found to the north, east, and south, but in fewer numbers and varieties. The rattlesnake is the only venomous snake native to California, but other venomous snakes make their home in the deserts of the American Southwest.

SYMPTOMS

Within 15 minutes to an hour after being bitten, the victim may begin to feel pain and notice swelling at the bite site. As time progresses, thirst, nausea and vomiting, muscle weakness, and shock may occur, depending on the type of rattlesnake. In cases of severe poisoning, the pain and swelling can become intense, blood pressure may drop, the pulse may become fast, and bleeding and bruising may begin to develop at sites remote from the bite.

EASTERN DIAMONDBACK

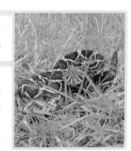

The eastern diamondback (also called the Florida diamondback) is considered to be one of the most deadly snakes in North America, with highly toxic venom. Heavier than its western relative and the largest of all venomous snakes in the United States—growing between five and seven feet long — the eastern diamondback has large dark brown or black diamonds with light centers on a body of olive, brown, or black. This snake can be aggressive, and is typically found in sparse woodland, dry pine flat woods, abandoned farms, and lowland coastal regions of the southeastern Gulf States.

WESTERN DIAMONDBACK

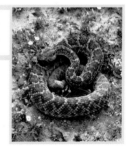

The western diamondback is one of the largest rattlers in the North American West, often reaching more than six feet in length. It has a heavy body and a large, spade-shaped head that is distinct from the neck. This snake is gray brown or pink, with light-bordered, dark diamond blotches on the back. The diamonds are often covered with small dark spots, and the distinctive tail is ringed boldly with black and white. This snake lives in semi-dry and dry arid areas, rocky canyons, river bluffs, and cultivated areas in the Southwest, and can be found as far south as central Mexico. It's found especially along the Colorado River. Toxicologists consider this snake to be one of the most dangerous in the United States.

TIMBER RATTLER

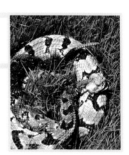

The timber rattler (*Crotalus horridus*) is the only rattlesnake found in populated areas of the northeastern United States, but its range extends into many of the central and southern states (except Florida). Three to four feet long, the timber rattler is the largest venomous snake in New York. The timber rattler in the northern range lives in pine forests and on wooded slopes. With a flat unmarked head and rough scales, this snake has a yellow brown or dark brown body, although completely black timber rattlers aren't uncommon.

CANEBRAKE RATTLER

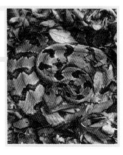

The canebrake rattler (*C. horridus atricaudatus*) is a type of timber rattler found in southern lowlands in cane thickets and swamps. The only noticeable difference between the canebrake and its cousin the timber rattler is that the canebrake has a rust-colored stripe down its back.

PACIFIC RATTLER

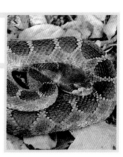

The Pacific rattler inhabits a variety of places in California and the Pacific northwest, from the Pacific Ocean to the inland valleys and desert areas, and up into the mountains above 10,000 feet. In southern California, the Pacific rattler shares a territory with several other species. This snake typically grows to between three and five feet long, and is more slender than the heavy-bodied eastern diamondback. The color of the Pacific rattler and its pattern of markings vary, with brown to grayish or greenish tones, and large blotches of lighter hues along its back.

MOJAVE RATTLER

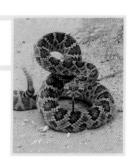

The Mojave rattler, found in the deserts of southeastern California, is the most venomous of any rattler in the United States. Growing up to four feet long, the Mojave rattler has dark diamond-shaped blotches on a greenish body and a distinct tail with white and black bands.

SIDEWINDER

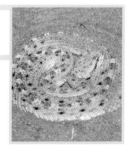

The small, yet venomous, sidewinder, also known as the horned rattlesnake, moves with a curious S-shaped sideways slither. It lives throughout the Mojave and

SNAKES

Sonoran deserts of southeastern California, western Arizona, southern Nevada, and extreme southwestern Utah. In addition to the arid desert flatlands, the sidewinder can be found in sandy washes, hardpan flats, and rocky areas below 5,000 feet.

The sidewinder is light tan, cream, pink, gray, or sandy, with darker patches on its back of gray, yellow, or tan, and a dark eye strip along its head. Mature adults are 18 to 32 inches in length. Fatalities are rare from this snake's bite.

COPPERHEAD

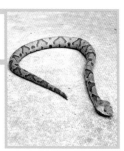

The distinctive copperhead, which gets its name from its dusky flame-colored head, is a member of the *Viperidae* family, a venomous species found in swampy, rocky, and wooded regions of eastern and central United States. Typically less than three feet long, the copperhead is a pink or red snake with a distinctive copper head and brown-red hourglass-shaped cross bands on its back. Although many bites are reported, the venom of this snake is less toxic than that of other snakes.

SYMPTOMS

A bite from this snake is usually followed by progressive swelling and pain at the site where the venom entered and started to spread. Copperhead bites are rarely associated with bleeding problems.

CORAL SNAKES

These beautiful but highly venomous snakes are twice as deadly as the rattlesnake, but are much less likely to bite. Just two types are found in the United States: the eastern and western varieties.

EASTERN CORAL SNAKE

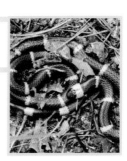

The eastern, or harlequin, coral snake lives in the southeastern United States. It's a burrowing snake with a small, blunt head and a cylindrical body, averaging 30 inches in length. While the body is ringed with bands of black, red, and yellow, the tail has yellow and black rings only.

WESTERN CORAL SNAKE

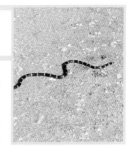

The western, or Sonoran, coral snake is a rather rare species found in the southwestern United States, and only grows to about 18 inches. It has much broader bands of yellow than those of its eastern cousin. You can tell the difference between the poisonous coral and a host of harmless similarly colored snakes by one specific detail of the coral's coloring: It's the only one with red bands touching yellow ones.

SYMPTOMS

The venom of coral snakes, like that of cobras, attacks the nervous system and causes paralysis. Because the coral snake must hold on tight to deliver its venom, it is less likely to cause a fatal wound. In addition, people rarely encounter coral snakes because they tend to burrow, and they seldom bite unless picked up.

TOADS

Snakes aren't the only poisonous creatures lurking out there. For families living in one limited geographical area, at least, there's another hazard that could come as a total surprise. And in this case, we're not talking about a bite!

Toads are part of the frog family but should not be mistaken for one. Unlike frogs, which have bulging eyes and slimy skin, toads have stubby bodies and dry skin. Their poison glands are behind their eyes. They have short hind legs for walking (instead of hopping, like a frog).

BUFO TOAD

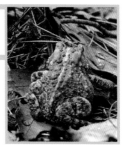

As big as a dinner plate and homely to boot, bufo toads all secrete toxic venom contained in glands behind their eyes at the base of the skull. The only Bufo found in the United States is the biggest one—the marine toad (*Bufo marinus*)—which was introduced into southern Florida. Like something out of a 1950s horror movie, today this giant toad lumbers across the Florida landscape in search of insects. While the Bufo is not aggressive, its secretions can poison a child curious or foolhardy enough to handle one carelessly.

Although these toads are available in pet stores in Florida, experts warn that there are far better—and safer—choices for companionship. While capable of killing any small dog foolish enough to try to bite it, the marine toads taste so unpleasant that most dogs immediately spit them out.

Bufo marine toads currently are established in southeastern Florida and the Tampa Bay area, but they are native to an area extending from Mexico and Central America to the Amazon Basin. They prefer developed areas, where they use man-made canals and ponds for spawning. Too large and slow to flee predators, the toads defend themselves by secreting their milky toxin.

PREVENTION!

You should make sure your children avoid these toads. If there is any physical contact, hands should be washed thoroughly. Homeowners can contact nuisance-animal trapping services to remove bufo toads.

SYMPTOMS

The toad's toxic secretion is most dangerous if swallowed, as some small dogs have discovered. It also can irritate a child's eyes and mucus membranes, and may cause allergic skin reactions in some people.

WHAT TO DO

Immediately wash affected skin with water and soap. If secretions get into the eye, they can cause extreme pain; immediately wash out your child's eyes with water or saline solution.

TOADS

5

DON'T GET STUNG

DANGEROUS INSECTS

It's the rare boy or girl who makes it through childhood without getting bitten by a tick, spider, or mosquito, or stung by a bee or scorpion. You can minimize your child's day-to-day risk by taking some preventive measures. It's also important to know what to do when the almost inevitable occurs.

BEES AND WASPS

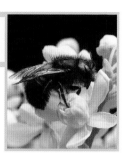

Stinging insects include wasps and bees, of the order *Hymenoptera*. While they may be widely feared, the idea that these insects are instinctively aggressive at any time and place is wrong, and blinds us to the vital role they play in nature. Although they can be an annoyance, stinging insects include species essential for pollinating fruits, vegetables, and flowers. Others are important predators of pest insects that infest both wild and cultivated plants. Still, there are risks associated with these stinging insects.

The two greatest problems from most insect stings are allergic reaction (which, in some individuals, can be fatal) and infection. It's wise to remember that bee stings cause up to four times as many deaths in the United States as do snakebites—not because bees are more venomous, but because so many people are allergic to bee stings. In fact, between one and two million people in the United States are severely allergic to the inflammatory substances in the venom of bees and wasps. This means the venom from a past sting has sensitized them, so that a single subsequent sting could provoke a severe allergic reaction that might be fatal. Since the bee venom's toxicity depends on the sensitivity of the victim and not on the venom itself, there is no bee antivenin available.

The different kinds of stinging insects that many people lump together as "bees" are not all alike. Hornets and yellow jackets are wasps that usually do not attack unless their nest is threatened, but they are the most lethal—grumpy, quick-tempered, and aggressive. In fact, they are so aggressive that they sting *and* bite at the same time. Yellow jackets have long, slender abdomens with yellow and black stripes. Hornets are reddish brown and yellow. The docile, lumbering honeybee has a round, smooth abdomen, but it's dwarfed by the even larger furry bumblebee.

Bees and wasps also sting differently. Wasps are able to extract their stinger and fly away, but the bee's stinger is often embedded in the skin, which means the poison sac and stinger are ripped out of the insect's abdomen; this is fatal to the bee.

PREVENTION!

There are several ways you can protect yourself and your family from being stung. Even before your children leave the house, they can lessen their chances of being stung by:

- Wearing clean clothes, and covering as much of their bodies as possible with clothing.

- Bathing daily.

Once outdoors, there are additional steps you can take to lessen the risk of stings. If bees are a problem for your family:

- Avoid setting out pots of flowering plants near the places where your family gathers. Bees hang around flowering plants.

- Check for new nests during the warmer hours of the day in July, August, and September, when bees and wasps are very active. Look in trees, in the corners of buildings, and in the ground where kids may play.

- Keep your home's outdoor areas clean, and keep picnic tables, grills, and other outdoor food sites neat.

- Listen for buzzing indicating a nest or swarm of bees or wasps, and be careful when entering sheds or outbuildings where bees may nest.

- Examine the work area before using lawn mowers, weed cutters, or other power equipment.

* Check out areas before tying up or penning pets or livestock.

* Urge kids to stay alert for bees and wasps while participating in all outdoor sports and activities.

* Never disturb a nest or swarm of bees or wasps; contact a pest control company or an emergency response organization instead.

HOW TO BEE-PROOF YOUR HOUSE

Follow these guidelines to protect your home from stinging insects.

* Inspect the outside walls and eaves of your home and outbuildings periodically for nests.

* Have nests removed from your house and yard as soon as they are discovered.

* Seal any openings bigger than $\frac{1}{8}$-inch in walls and around chimneys and plumbing.

* Install $\frac{1}{8}$-inch hardware cloth as a screen over the tops of rain spouts, vents, and openings in water meters and utility boxes.

* From spring through fall, check for bees entering or leaving the same area of your home or yard; pay particular attention along the ground.

 WHAT TO DO IN AN ATTACK
Most stinging insects will not attack if left alone. If provoked, however, a bee or wasp will sting in defense of its nest or itself.

If bees or wasps are in the area, there are several ways to lessen an attack:

⊗ If a single stinging insect is flying around, remain still or cover your face, which is the most likely place for a bee or wasp to sting.

⊗ Don't swing or swat at an insect—it may provoke it to sting.

⊗ If attacked by several stinging insects at the same time, run! Bees release a chemical when they sting that alerts other bees to the intruder. More bees often follow.

⊗ If attacked by a swarm of bees, run indoors or to an outdoor, shaded area.

⊗ If a bee gets into the car, slowly pull off the road and open all the windows.

BEE PROBLEMS: WHOM TO CALL

For a sting emergency: Call 911.

For honeybee swarms or hives outdoors: Call your local Environmental Health Department.

For swarms or hives inside the house: Call a licensed pest control company.

SYMPTOMS OF A STING

The area around a bee sting will get red, swell, and cause pain, which can last for about 24 hours. More widespread reactions include swelling and redness of the entire limb where the sting occurred. The more severe, systemic (body-wide) reactions in-

BEES/WASPS

clude hives, itching, swelling, low blood pressure, difficulty breathing, and anaphylactic shock (a severe reaction involving most or all of these symptoms).

If you get stung on the forehead and your eyelids swell, it means you are having a local reaction. But if you get stung on the toe and your eyelids swell, then you are having a systemic reaction. Widespread local reactions aren't usually serious and rarely indicate that you'll have a severe allergic reaction in the future. However, a systemic allergic reaction means your body is sending you a warning, and this could indicate that the next sting you get will involve equally (or even more) serious reactions.

Anyone who is stung multiple times can have a fourth type of reaction called a toxic reaction. This is not an allergic reaction, but is a direct result of getting a large dose of bee venom. Symptoms can include fever, weakness, nausea, vomiting, and pain. Although these toxic reactions are rarely serious, they may sensitize a person to future stings, which could indicate future allergic reactions may occur.

WHAT TO DO FOR A STING

If your child has been stung by a bee or wasp, follow these guidelines:

* If a bee has left behind its stinger attached to a venom sac, don't try to pull it out, which could squeeze the sac and release more venom. Instead, gently scrape it out with a credit card or dull knife.

* Wash the area of the sting carefully with soap and water.

* Apply ice wrapped in a cloth over the area.

* To ease the pain, apply a paste of baking soda and water to the site and leave it on for 15 to 20 minutes.

✕ For additional pain relief, give acetaminophen (Tylenol).

✕ Administer an over-the-counter antihistamine if approved by the doctor. Be sure to follow correct children's dosage instructions.

✕ Have an adult stay with the victim to watch out for an allergic reaction.

STING EMERGENCY!

Call **911** and seek medical help immediately if your child:

✕ Is stung inside the mouth or nose, because swelling may block airways quickly.

✕ Has large areas of swelling in parts of the body other than the sting site.

✕ Is having trouble breathing, is breathing abnormally, or is wheezing.

✕ Feels a tightness in throat or chest.

✕ Is dizzy.

✕ Develops hives.

✕ Faints.

✕ Experiences continuous nausea and vomiting.

Because allergic reactions to insect stings can be rapidly fatal, people with known allergies to stings should always carry an insect sting allergy kit containing self-injectable epinephrine, and wear a medical ID bracelet or necklace describing their allergy. Your doctor can give you information about the allergy kit.

BEES/WASPS

AFRICANIZED "KILLER BEES"

Africanized honey bees, popularly known as "killer bees," developed when African bees brought to Brazil in 1956 escaped and mated with European honeybees. Since then, they have gradually spread north through South America, Central America, and Mexico, traveling about 100 miles a year. They landed in southern Texas in 1990, Arizona in 1993, and California two years later. They are expected to continue to form colonies in parts of the South.

Africanized bees look like the common honeybee, but they are very dangerous. They attack in groups, although each bee only can sting once. Since their introduction into Brazil, they have killed more than 1,000 people. Africanized bees are extremely volatile and have been known to chase an intended victim for a quarter of a mile. They are also able to sense a threat from people or animals 50 feet or more from the nest, and they can detect vibrations 100 feet away.

If you get in the way of killer bees, follow the steps on page 129. And follow these extra steps:

✳ Cover your face and head, which is the target for these bees, with a towel, handkerchief, blanket, or jacket. If you don't have anything else, pull your shirt up over your face. Stings to your torso will be less serious than stings to your face.

✳ Run indoors. Do *not* jump into a lake, pond, or pool, because the bees will simply wait for you to come up for air and sting your face and head.

✳ Once you're safe, call 911 immediately if you've been stung.

CATERPILLARS

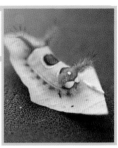

Many parents have no idea that there are eight types of caterpillars that can pack a painful sting if a child innocently touches one. All caterpillars are larvae (the "worm" form of insects). While all of them seem fuzzy and harmless, some types of caterpillars possess sharp, stinging hairs. These are either hollow and connected to poison glands (so that venom flows on contact), or similar to glass fibers that break off easily in skin, causing a needle-prick pain.

Toxic caterpillars don't deliberately attack the way wasps or bees do. Stings typically occur when a child accidentally brushes against one of these caterpillars, or tries to pick up one by hand. Such incidents usually occur in late summer to early autumn, when these caterpillars are generally found on corn leaves, vegetable plants, shrubs, and trees.

PREVENTION!

These caterpillars can drop out of trees onto a person, crawl into clothing on the ground, or sting when brushed against. Be careful when trying to brush one of these caterpillars off, and never swat or crush one by hand. Instead, remove it carefully and slowly with a stick or other object. It's a good idea to warn your children about handling or playing with any colorful, hairy, or fuzzy caterpillar, since it may be difficult to distinguish between harmless and venomous insect larvae.

Never pick up hairy, fuzzy, or spiny caterpillars by hand except with heavy leather gloves. Wear long-sleeve shirts, pants, and gloves when harvesting sweet corn in late summer and early autumn to avoid possible stings.

These stinging hair caterpillars are not usually found in sufficient numbers to warrant the use of pesticide sprays. However, if you do have an infestation around your house, shrubs and trees can be sprayed to reduce or eliminate the caterpillars. Sprays of acephate (Orthene), carbaryl (Sevin), Diazinon, or chlorpyrifos (Dursban), in formulations labeled for bushes, shrubs, and trees, can be helpful. Be sure to read the label and follow all directions and safety precautions.

SYMPTOMS OF POISONING

Depending on the child and the caterpillar, reaction to a sting may range from reddening, swelling, burning, and itching, to severe pain at the site of the sting. Typically, following a caterpillar sting, inflammation, swelling, and numbness occur at or around the area of contact. More severe reactions to venom may lead to whole-body signs such as fever, nausea, vomiting, and headache.

Hypersensitive youngsters may experience severe swelling at the site of the sting and other reactions that might require hospital treatment. In some cases, poisonous caterpillar hairs can get into a child's eye and cause significant damage or even blindness.

The type of reaction depends on the species of caterpillar, degree of contact, type of toxin, and sensitivity. Reactions may be especially severe for children with allergies or sensitive skin. There is also a chance that the caterpillar spines may break off in the skin, leading to a foreign body reaction and potential risk of secondary bacterial infection.

Although the irritation is usually caused by direct contact with a live caterpillar, some species can retain stinging capabilities for some time after death. However, the reaction caused by contact with dead caterpillars, cast skins, or cocoons is generally milder than the sting of a live caterpillar.

WHAT TO DO

The key to limiting the sting from any of these caterpillars is to quickly and repeatedly apply adhesive or transparent tape over the sting site to remove the broken hairs or spines. Washing the affected skin area thoroughly with soap and water may help remove irritating venom.

Next, promptly apply an ice pack and a baking soda poultice to help reduce pain and swelling. (To make this poultice, add water to a few tablespoons of baking soda to make a paste.)

Painkillers such as acetaminophen don't work very well in easing the pain and headache caused by these stings, but over-the-counter oral antihistamines may help relieve itching and burning. Topical corticosteroids may reduce the intensity of the inflammatory reaction.

You should call 911 or get to the hospital emergency room if a severe reaction is evident. Infants, toddlers, and those in poor health are more likely to suffer serious reaction symptoms, as are children with asthma or severe allergies.

The eight varieties of toxic caterpillars include:

✳ Buck moth caterpillar (*Hemileuca maia*)
✳ Hagmoth caterpillar (*Phobetron pithecium*)
✳ Hickory tussock or hickory tiger caterpillar (*Lophocampa caryae*)
✳ Io caterpillar (*Automeris io*)
✳ Puss caterpillar (*Megalopyge opercularis*)
✳ Saddleback caterpillar (*Sibine stimulea*)
✳ Silverspotted tiger caterpillar (*Halisidota argentata*)
✳ Stinging rose caterpillar (*Parasa indetermina*)

BUCK MOTH CATERPILLAR

SCIENTIFIC NAME
Hemileuca maia

These larvae are similar in size and appearance to those of the io moth, but the colors range from purple to black with lots of small pale yellow dots scattered over the body. They are covered with reddish to black branches and stinging spines. The forelegs are red and the true legs are glossy black. Adults fly in late September and early October, with peak moth activity coinciding with the rutting season of whitetail deer (hence the name). The tiny larvae winter inside egg cases, emerging in late spring and summer. The caterpillars feed on oak and willow trees.

HAGMOTH CATERPILLAR

SCIENTIFIC NAME
Phobetron pithecium

Sometimes called the monkey slug, this caterpillar is distinctive in form and easy to identify. These brownish larvae are about $5/8$ inch long when full grown, with long black stinging hairs that curve and twist, vaguely resembling the messy hairdo of a hag (or witch)—thus the name. Hagmoth caterpillars feed on various shrubs and lower branches of ornamental trees.

HICKORY TUSSOCK CATERPILLAR OR HICKORY TIGER CATERPILLAR

SCIENTIFIC NAME
Lophocampa caryae

This toxic caterpillar, which goes by two names, comes in different colors. Some are white-haired with black spots clearly seen on each body segment, whereas others are furry and white with a row of black, furry dots down the back and two long, black tufts of hair near the coal-black head. When fully grown, caterpillars are about $1^{1}/_{2}$ inches long. Moths appear in May through July;

CATERPILLARS

eggs are laid in clusters of 100 or more on the undersides of leaves. Young larvae feed gregariously, later scattering to feed. The caterpillars require about three months to develop, and cocoons are built on or near the ground in late September and early October. You'll find these caterpillars in walnut, hickory, butternut, apple, basswood, birch, elm, black locust, aspen, and linden trees.

Although the hickory tussock is not always officially listed as a stinging type, there are verified reports of schoolchildren developing skin rashes and itching after playing with these caterpillars. The rash looks a lot like poison ivy, and may cause a severe itch followed by a painful burning sensation.

IO MOTH CATERPILLAR

SCIENTIFIC NAME
Automeris io

These pale-green larvae are 2 to 2$\frac{1}{2}$ inches long when full grown. Extending lengthwise along each side of the body is a narrow reddish stripe edged below with white. Each body segment is equipped with several fleshy knobs armed with numerous long, greenish venomous spines tipped with black. The sting is less severe than that of the puss caterpillar.

Io moth larvae are general feeders, and can be found on corn foliage, cotton, roses, and a wide variety of trees and shrubs, including apple, black locust, cherry, dogwood, elm, hackberry, hickory, maple, oak, sycamore, and willow. Scientists believe they only reproduce once a year. Larvae winter inside a tough oval cocoon, often enclosed in leaves on the ground. Moths emerge in the spring and summer, then mate and lay eggs.

CATERPILLARS

PUSS CATERPILLAR

SCIENTIFIC NAME
Megalopyge opercularis

The sting of a puss caterpillar is considered to be the most severe of all the stinging caterpillars. These larvae, about one inch long when full grown, are broad and somewhat flat (pear-shaped) with a dense covering of silky gray to reddish-brown hairs. Interspersed among the long body hairs are lots of short spines that discharge venom on contact. Hairs peak roof-like over the back and taper rearward to form a "tail." Hairs along the ridge of the back occur in small tufts; on each side are small patches of white.

Moths emerge from their cocoons in late spring and early summer, when they mate and deposit eggs on trees and shrubs. The eggs hatch in a few days, and the caterpillar matures a few weeks after that. You'll find these toxic fellows on broadleaf shrubs such as hackberry, oak, maple, sycamore, elm, English ivy, rose, and other plants.

SADDLEBACK CATERPILLAR

SCIENTIFIC NAME
Sibine stimulea

This caterpillar (pictured on page 133) is particularly problematic, since it tends to attract curious youngsters fascinated by its bright neon-green color and a dark brown to black "saddle." The "saddle" looks like an oval purplish-brown spot in the middle of a green patch on its back. Children sometimes find saddleback caterpillars around shrubs and get stung by handling them. About an inch long, the caterpillar has poisonous spines on four large projections, and many smaller ones on the sides of its body. The hollow poisonous hairs are connected to underlying poison glands.

You'll find this brown and green larva of the moth *Sibine stimulea* on shade trees and ornamental shrubs throughout the eastern United States in late summer—especially on the leaves of basswood, chestnut, cherry, plum, and oak. Fortunately, saddleback caterpillars tend to be loners; just because you find one in your backyard doesn't necessarily mean others will be lurking nearby.

SILVERSPOTTED TIGER MOTH CATERPILLAR

SCIENTIFIC NAME
Halisidota argentata

This caterpillar, about 1 to 1½ inches long when full-grown, is covered with dense tufts of brown or black poisonous hairs. Stings can be rather painful. After emerging in July and August, the caterpillar feeds on Douglas fir, true fir, pine, and other conifers. Feeding occurs in clusters under a web formed with dead needles where wintering occurs. Larvae disperse the following spring, feeding singly until they mature. These caterpillars spin cocoons of silk and body hairs, attaching them to twigs, needles, tree trunks, or litter on the forest floor.

STINGING ROSE CATERPILLAR

SCIENTIFIC NAME
Parasa indetermina

This slug-like caterpillar is about an inch long with narrow black stripes edged with yellow extending lengthwise along each side of the body. There are four black stripes lengthwise down the back, with 12 pale-yellow knobs armed with spines. Other clusters of spines on orange-red knobs appear along each side.

A useful identifying feature is the broad purplish band down the midline of the back. Within the band are narrow, whitish longitudinal lines, which may be interrupted by constrictions. The stinging rose is similar in habits to the hagmoth, wintering in a cocoon on the ground. They are usually found in August. Hosts of the stinging rose caterpillar include rose bushes and apple, cottonwood, dogwood, hickory, oak, redbud, and sycamore trees.

TICKS

These tiny, bloodsucking pests were once considered to be simply an annoying irritation that plagued dogs and cats more than their owners—until the discovery that some varieties cause a range of diseases including Rocky Mountain spotted fever, babesiosis, ehrlichiosis, and Lyme disease, now epidemic in the Northeast. There are more than 200 species of ticks in the United States that frequent woods, lawns, beach grass—and also urban areas. Unlike fleas, ticks are not truly insects, but arachnids, as are mites, spiders, and scorpions.

DEER TICKS

Ticks that cause Lyme disease are most likely found in coastal states from Maine to Maryland, in the upper Midwest, and on the Pacific coast. They are most common in wet weather in late spring or early summer, although they may appear whenever the temperature is above 40 degrees F. for several consecutive days. About half of all deer ticks in the Northeast carry a type of bacteria called *Borrelia burgdorferi* that causes Lyme disease. (On Nantucket, Massachusetts, and Block Island, Rhode Island, however, the percentage of disease-carrying ticks is much higher.) These ticks are so tiny that anyone who is bitten may never notice its presence. The tick must be attached to a person for between 36 and 48 hours before the bacteria are transmitted. Most infections can be avoided by carefully checking yourself and your children for ticks every day.

The tick that transmits Lyme disease in California relies on intermediate hosts such as lizards that are resistant to infection. For this reason, ticks in the West (and, consequently, people in that region) are much less often infected.

PREVENTION!

There is a Lyme disease vaccine for dogs, but a vaccine developed for humans was recalled. Experts at the National Centers for Disease Control and Prevention (CDC) do not recommend preventive treatment with antibiotics after every tick bite; they believe it is better to prevent bites in the first place. When walking in the woods, make sure to stay on trails and avoid brushing up against tall grass where ticks are liable to be clinging. Ticks don't hop, jump, fly, or descend from trees—but they can blow in a strong breeze.

To prevent bites, the entire family should wear protective clothing—light-colored, long-sleeved shirts or blouses, with light-colored pants tucked into boots or socks. Light-colored clothes allow "stowaway" ticks to be more easily spotted.

An insect repellent with DEET (N, N-diethyl-meta-toluamide) may be used on bare skin and clothing; Duranon can be applied to clothing only (not to skin). Any insect repellent should be used with caution on children, and should not be applied to their hands or face.

Because ticks and their hosts (mice, chipmunks, voles, and

TICKS

other small mammals) need moisture and a good hiding place away from direct sun, the cleaner the area around your house the better. Remove all leaf litter and brush as far as possible from your house, and prune low-lying bushes to let in more sun. Rake up leaves quickly, since ticks prefer to winter in leaves. Woodpiles are another favorite hiding place for mammals carrying ticks, so keep your wood off the ground, in a sunny place, under cover, and far from your house.

Clean up your garden each fall, and get rid of foliage on the ground that could provide winter shelter for mammals carrying ticks. Stone walls also increase the potential for ticks. Because even shady lawns support ticks in epidemic areas, mow and edge your lawn carefully. Entire fields of brush should be mowed in the fall.

Because birdfeeders may attract birds that have ticks, don't put feeders too close to the house, and clean up the ground under the feeder regularly. Stop feeding birds in late spring and summer, when infected ticks are most active. Building eight-foot fences to keep out deer can significantly reduce the number of ticks in an area. If you allow your pets outside each day, you should regularly check them for ticks and apply flea and tick repellent monthly.

SYMPTOMS OF POISONING

A typical tick bite causes no pain but usually triggers an annoying itch. Those ticks that carry Lyme disease, however, may cause an additional large red rash radiating outward from the bite, sometimes with a telltale "bulls-eye" white center. Between three days and a month after being infected, up to 60 percent of victims will notice this red rash. But remember—this means that 40 percent won't notice any skin symptoms at all!

As the bacteria move through the body, other reactions may occur, including such flu-like symptoms as stiff neck, headache, appetite loss, body aches, and fatigue. Lyme disease symptoms tend to persist or recur, which differentiates it from the flu. Early neurological problems may appear in about 20 percent of victims, including numbness or tingling in various parts of the body.

If untreated, about half of those who get bitten develop recurrent attacks of painful, swollen joints that last for weeks to months. This arthritis-like pain may shift from one joint to another, but the knee is most often affected. Between 10 and 20 percent of untreated Lyme patients will go on to develop chronic Lyme arthritis. Unlike other types of arthritis, Lyme arthritis may not affect both sides of the body equally. One out of 10 Lyme patients develop heart problems, which aren't usually obvious unless a physician picks up the telltale signs. Other symptoms can include memory loss, concentration problems, and changes in mood or sleeping habits. Pregnant women who contract Lyme disease have a higher risk of miscarriage, stillbirth, or delivering an infant with birth defects.

Some experts believe that a small number of appropriately treated patients with Lyme disease will experience a recurrence of symptoms a few years after the initial infection, especially if their immune system has been temporarily suppressed (such as by taking certain medicines, or having a vaccination). Recurrence requires another round of antibiotic treatment.

WHAT TO DO

Ticks secrete a cement-like substance that helps them adhere firmly to the skin, so if your child has been bitten, you shouldn't just yank the tick out of the skin. It is important to remove it properly: Using fine-point tweezers, grasp the tick as close to the skin as possible and gently pull it straight out. Dispose of the tick, then wash your hands and the bite site. Write down the date and the location on the body where the tick bite occurred, and then call your doctor to determine if treatment is necessary. Watch the bite site and then continue to monitor your child's general health for signs or symptoms of a tick-borne illness.

AT THE DOCTOR'S OFFICE

If a red rash or other symptoms of Lyme disease develop, antibiotic treatment must begin as soon as possible. Antibiotics (doxycycline, tetracycline, or amoxicillin) begun within three days of a tick bite should ensure complete recovery, but most people treated in later stages respond well too. Some cases that aren't diagnosed early may resist antibiotic therapy, leading to persistent infection.

WHAT NOT TO DO WITH A TICK

✖ Don't touch the tick with your bare hands. If you must remove it with your fingers, use a tissue or leaf to avoid touching infected tick fluids.

✖ Don't try to remove a tick by pricking it, crushing it, or touching it with a hot match; this may cause the tick to release infected fluids or tissue.

✖ Don't try to smother the tick by painting it with petroleum jelly or nail polish; the tick has enough oxygen to complete feeding.

MOSQUITOES

Until recent years, the bite of a mosquito was seen as a simple annoyance in modern malaria-free North America. But mosquito bites have become much more serious in the wake of the emergence of West Nile virus (WNV) in the United States. Experts believe WNV is now established as a seasonal epidemic that flares up in the summer and continues into the fall. The virus is transmitted to humans via the bite of mosquitoes that become infected when they feed on infected birds. When a mosquito bites you or your child, the virus may be injected. It multiplies in the blood and then moves into the brain, where it can inflame brain tissue and affect the central nervous system.

However, even in areas where mosquitoes carry the virus, fewer than 1 percent are infected. And less than 1 percent of people bitten and infected by an WNV-carrying mosquito become severely ill. The virus is not spread by touching or kissing a person who has the disease, or from a health care worker who has treated someone with the disease.

PREVENTION!

The easiest way to avoid the disease is to prevent mosquito bites. Mosquitoes are generally most active at dusk and dawn, so be sure to use insect repellent and have your kids wear long sleeves and pants at these times—or keep them indoors during these hours. Wear light colors to help detect them on your clothes. Insect repellents containing DEET (N, N-diethyl-meta-toluamide) are by far the best. DEET comes in various strengths, but the more concentrated, the more effective. Use weaker strengths on children because heavy doses can be toxic. Repellent should not be applied directly to hands or the face. Although many consumers swear by Avon's Skin-so-Soft, research by the military as well as by Avon has demonstrated it is not as effective as DEET.

To keep mosquitoes out of your home, maintain the screens on your windows and doors. Eliminate mosquito-breeding sites by draining standing water anywhere on your property, including in flowerpot liners, buckets, and barrels. Change the water in pet dishes frequently and replace the water in birdbaths weekly (or use a pump on your bird bath to keep water moving). Drill holes in tire swings so water drains out. Empty children's wading pools

MOSQUITOES

after each use and store them on their sides.

While there is no evidence that a person can get the virus from handling live or dead infected birds, barehanded contact should be avoided. If you need to handle any dead animal, use gloves or double plastic bags to place the carcass in a garbage can.

SYMPTOMS OF POISONING

About four out of five people who are infected with West Nile virus won't have any symptoms at all. Up to 20 percent of those infected may develop symptoms, such as fever, headache, body aches, nausea and vomiting, and occasionally swollen lymph glands or a skin rash on the chest, stomach, and back. These symptoms can last for just a few days or several weeks.

About one in 150 people infected with West Nile virus develop severe illness characterized by high fever, headache, neck stiffness, stupor, disorientation, coma, tremors, convulsions, muscle weakness, vision loss, numbness, and paralysis. These symptoms may last several weeks, and neurological effects may be permanent. The fatality rate from severe illness ranges from 3 to 15 percent.

WEST NILE VIRUS AND BLOOD TRANSFUSIONS

All donated blood is checked for West Nile. The risk of getting WNV through blood transfusions or organ transplants is very small and should not prevent anyone who needs blood from having a transfusion. If you're worried, talk to your doctor.

WHO'S AT RISK FOR WEST NILE?

Mosquitoes carrying this virus can infect anyone, but there are a few groups of people who are at higher risk for developing severe disease. These include:

✖ **People over age 50.** These individuals should take special care to avoid bites, since they are more likely to develop serious symptoms if they become infected.

✖ **People who frequent the outdoors.** The more time you and your family spend outside at dusk when mosquitoes are active, the higher your chance of being bitten.

WHAT TO DO

Wash any mosquito bite with soap and water, and then apply an antiseptic. To control itching, you can use a nonprescription topical antihistamine, calamine lotion, anesthetic gel, or ice pack. Alternatively, a paste of water and baking soda can be applied. Milder symptoms of West Nile should improve without treatment; you don't need to seek medical attention. However, symptoms of severe illness, such as unusually severe headaches or confusion, require immediate medical attention and possibly hospitalization. Pregnant women and nursing mothers are encouraged to consult their doctor if they develop symptoms of West Nile virus.

AT THE HOSPITAL

There is no specific treatment for West Nile infection. In more severe cases, hospitalized patients will receive intravenous fluids, help with breathing, and nursing care.

MOSQUITOES

SPIDERS

You may be unnerved to learn that most of the 50,000 species of spiders in the United States actually have poison glands connected to their fangs. But only a few are capable of piercing human skin, and only two—the black widow and the brown recluse—are significantly toxic to people. Generally speaking, most spider attacks occur when someone disturbs a nest while working outside.

BLACK WIDOW SPIDER

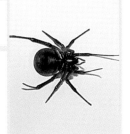

One of only two truly poisonous spiders found in the United States, the black widow has a shiny black body with an orange or red hourglass marking on its belly (some spiders have a spot instead of an hourglass). Male spiders, which aren't considered dangerous, are much smaller than females, typically brown, and may only have a little red dot.

Although all six species of black widow spider are venomous, bites are rarely fatal.

Their messy webs are often found under or between rocks, around outdoor water faucets, and in woodpiles, garages, basements, garbage cans, and sheds. Black widows are found throughout the United States and Canada, but most live in warmer climates.

PREVENTION!

Be very careful about letting children play around areas where black widow spiders may live. If you're working in such an area, wear gloves and be attentive. This spider is resistant to many insecticides. To eradicate the black widow, remove all materials where these spiders might hide, knock down the webs and their round egg sacs with a stick, and crush them underfoot. Destroying the egg sacs helps control the population.

SYMPTOMS OF POISONING

The actual bite of the black widow isn't especially painful—it might not be felt at all. There may be a bit of swelling with two tiny puncture marks, followed by a dull numbing pain that gets worse as time passes. The pain peaks within three hours, but continues for another two days.

Within 40 minutes after the bite, the venom begins to attack nerves, causing muscles to tighten—first at the location of the bite and then progressing to involve the abdominal or chest muscles. At the same time, there may be abdominal cramps, nausea, vomiting, fever, chills, palpitations, high blood pressure, wheezing or difficult breathing, sweating, convulsions, and delirium. Most patients, however, recover without complication.

WHAT TO DO

Cleanse the wound, keep the victim warm and quiet, and apply a cool compress over the bite location. Keep the affected limb elevated above heart level. Tylenol may be used to relieve minor symptoms. Call a doctor or the regional Poison Control Center (1-800-222-1222) right away.

AT THE HOSPITAL

Antivenin is available, but most patients can be managed without it. Healthy people typically recover rapidly in one to five days. However, children under age 16 or people over age 60, especially those with a heart condition, may require a hospital stay. A tetanus shot may be needed.

SPIDERS

BROWN RECLUSE SPIDER

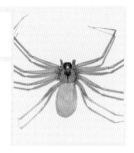

The other toxic spider found in the United States is the brown recluse. Native to Central and South America, the brown recluse is believed to have been accidentally imported into this country in fruit or vegetable crates at some point during the past 50 years. Since then, it's been steadily moving north and west, and now ranges from Texas and Arkansas to as far north as Massachusetts.

This brown, half-inch-long spider has a dark violin-shaped mark on its back and is typically found indoors, spinning webs in dark corners. Brown recluses get their name from their habit of hiding in dresser drawers and closets (often in folds of clothing), garages, attics, and sheds. They won't try to bite unless they are trapped. The venom of the female is more potent than that of the male.

SYMPTOMS OF POISONING

The physical reaction to a brown recluse spider bite depends on how much venom was injected and the victim's sensitivity to it. Some people are unaffected by a bite, whereas others experience immediate or delayed effects as the venom kills tissues at the wound site. Typically, most people don't feel much pain at first. But if a brown recluse bites your child, within eight hours the pain may become severe and the area will begin to turn red. Any area on the skin that the spider has bitten will begin to die and slough off, because the venom contains a substance that is very destructive to skin. This leads to a large, spreading sore that becomes a dark, hard blister within a few days. In some cases, this blister turns deep purple, and within two weeks becomes an open ulcer. For a small number of victims, the ulcer takes a very long time to heal.

In rare instances, the bite may cause a number of body-wide

reactions, including fever, chills, weakness, nausea and vomiting, joint pain, and rash. Fatal bites are exceedingly rare.

WHAT TO DO

Keep the victim calm and immediately contact your physician, hospital, or the regional Poison Control Center (1-800-222-1222). Apply an ice pack directly to the bite area to relieve swelling and pain. If possible, collect the spider in a plastic bag, small jar, or pill vial for identification.

AT THE HOSPITAL

There is no specific antivenin. The surgical removal of affected skin was once standard procedure, but now experts believe this slows down wound healing. Treatment with oral dapsone (an antibiotic used mainly for leprosy) has been suggested to reduce the degree of tissue damage, but evidence is scant that it is beneficial. Since effective treatments have not yet been found, treating the symptoms is the main option.

SCORPION

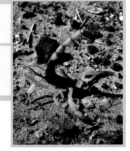

SCIENTIFIC NAME
Centruroides exilicauda

Looking a lot like a crab with extra legs, the scorpion is a relative of the spider, mite, and tick. There are about 1,300 species of scorpions worldwide; about 90 of those can be found in the United States, all but four living west of the Mississippi River.

Scorpions have elongated bodies and a segmented tail tipped with a venomous stinger that's so flexible it's almost impossible to pick one up in your bare hands without getting stung—a fact you should make very clear to your kids if you live in scorpion territory.

Despite the scorpion's scary reputation and creepy appearance, only one species in the United States has venom potent enough to be dangerous to humans—*Centruroides exilicauda* (formerly called *C. sculpturatus*), found in much of Arizona. A small population occurs in extreme southeastern California, and a few have crept into southern Utah and Nevada.

The scorpion of the American Southwest inflicts severe pain and is especially dangerous to children. The venom is a complex mixture of neurotoxins (poisons that affect the victim's nervous system) and other substances.

PREVENTION!

Scorpions don't chase and attack people, despite what you may have seen in the movies. But they will sting if picked up or stepped on. They prefer moist, dark places and often hide in clothing or shoes.

Scorpions are roaming hunters, and infested houses are usually the result of scorpions that find easy routes inside. Scorpions are tough to control with insecticides alone, so the best thing you can do is modify the area around your house. Move all trash, logs, boards, stones, and bricks away from the dwelling, and keep the grass closely mowed. Prune bushes and overhanging tree branches near the house, so they can't provide a handy way for scorpions to get to your roof. Store garbage cans off the ground, and never bring firewood inside the house unless you're putting it right onto the fire.

Install weather stripping around doors and windows (inside and out) and along baseboards. Plug any holes in the walls with steel wool, pieces of nylon scouring pad, or small squares of screen. Caulk eaves, pipes, and cracks, and make sure your window screens are in good repair and fitted tightly in the window frame.

Check your outdoor property with a fluorescent black light (also called a Wood's lamp) just after dark. If there are scorpions present, they will glow brightly in this light, helping you to determine how well established they are and where they are breeding. Homeowners with heavy infestations often set out a wet burlap sack at night; scorpions will crawl in and can then be easily located and destroyed in the morning. Residents in areas where scorpions are endemic should always shake out all shoes, bedding, and clothing before using.

SYMPTOMS OF POISONING

A scorpion sting produces severe pain and swelling at the site, much like a bee sting. The stung area may swell, become discolored, and even form a blister. These symptoms may last for 8 to 12 hours.

If the sting is from *C. exilicauda,* a pins-and-needles sensation may develop at the sting site. The area may not get swollen or discolored, but within one to three hours the victim may experience double vision, tightness of the jaw muscles, difficulty speaking, restlessness, numbness, frothing at the mouth, breathing problems (including respiratory paralysis), muscle twitching, painful spasms, nausea, vomiting, incontinence, drowsiness, irregular heartbeat, and—in rare instances—convulsions. Neurological symptoms that appear within two to four hours indicate a serious medical problem. Death is uncommon because toxicity is dose-related, but the smaller the victim, the higher the risk of a fatal sting.

WHAT TO DO

Medical attention is not always necessary. If a scorpion stings someone in your family, call the regional Poison Control Center (1-800-222-1222) immediately. Have the victim lie still, with the sting area immobile and lower than the heart. Apply ice packs to the wound. If pain is the only symptom, a cold compress and painkillers may be sufficient. You should not apply hot packs or alcohol, or make an incision over the sting.

AT THE HOSPITAL

An antivenin is available for severe stings of *C. exilicauda* scorpions. Anesthetics and painkillers may be administered if the pain is confined to the site of the bite.

6

DANGER—DON'T TOUCH!

CHEMICALS

Some of the most common poisoning problems in the home are caused by chemicals, pesticides, cleaners, gases, and chemically treated products—and an alarming number of those incidents involve children.

Far too many parents are remarkably relaxed about how and where they store poisonous insecticides, herbicides, and other household chemicals. A recent survey by the U.S. Environmental Protection Agency found that almost half of all households with children under the age of five had at least one pesticide stored in an unlocked cabinet less than four feet off the ground. The survey also found that 75 percent of households without children under age five stored pesticides within reach of kids. That's especially significant, since 13 percent of all pediatric pesticide poisonings occur in homes other than where the child lives. To keep your kids safe, be sure to follow these guidelines.

✳ Always store pesticides away from children's reach, in a locked cabinet or garden shed.

✳ Read the label of any chemical product first and always follow the directions, including all precautions and restrictions.

✳ Before applying pesticides or using other chemicals, make sure your kids and their toys are out of the area. Keep them away until the site is dry, or as recommended by the label.

✳ Never leave pesticides or other chemicals unattended when you're using them, not even for a few minutes.

✳ Never transfer pesticides or chemicals to other containers, jars, or cans; children may associate certain containers with food or drinks.

✳ Close the containers of all toxic products tightly after using them.

ALCOHOL

Even though drinking alcoholic beverages is safe for most people in moderation, it's important to keep in mind that alcohol is a chemical that in high doses can be extremely dangerous. Drinking too much alcohol can cause potentially fatal complications that require emergency medical treatment. Unfortunate examples are adolescent drinking rituals or hazings in which teenagers drink large amounts of beer or liquor as fast as they can. The result: Alcohol enters the bloodstream so quickly and rises to such levels that the liver can't metabolize it. The teenage drinker may lose consciousness, suffer heart or breathing problems, and even die.

Even in small amounts, alcohol can cause problems in young children. A curious toddler may discover an alcoholic beverage in a glass or container left by an adult, and drink it. This is especially common during the holidays when families are celebrating at homes other than their own, which may not be childproofed.

Accidental alcohol consumption can quickly lead to symptoms in young children due to their small size. In addition, youngsters are more susceptible to developing low blood sugar after drinking alcohol, which can lead to coma or seizures.

SYMPTOMS OF POISONING

Alcohol slows down the body's functions, decreasing heart and respiratory rates, and lowering blood pressure. Early symptoms of alcohol poisoning include cold, clammy, or bluish skin. Alcohol poisoning can cause liver and/or respiratory failure, which can affect the heart. As the vital body organs are deprived of oxygen, the victim can drift into unconsciousness, eventually suffer irreversible brain damage or even die.

CHEMICALS

WHAT TO DO

If you suspect someone has drunk too much alcohol and has lapsed into unconsciousness, try to wake him. If you can't seem to get a response, turn him onto his side so that possible vomiting won't block the airway. A person who is breathing irregularly —taking a few breaths and then pausing without breathing— may need medical attention. If the breathing rate is less than eight breaths a minute, or if more than 10 seconds pass between breaths, you should get help immediately. Call the regional Poison Control Center (1-800-222-1222) or dial 911. Monitor the person's breathing and make sure he doesn't roll onto his back.

Do *not* put anyone who has drunk too much alcohol into a cold shower—the shock of the cold can trigger loss of consciousness. Do not give a severely drunk person anything to eat or drink; this can cause vomiting or choking.

AT THE HOSPITAL

In cases of alcohol poisoning, emergency medical support can be life-saving. In the most severe cases, the intoxicated person may need to be placed on life support until the alcohol in the body is metabolized. Intravenous fluids and glucose may need to be administered.

ANTIFREEZE

Most types of automobile radiator antifreeze contain ethylene glycol. Because antifreeze tastes sweet, it may attract children as well as pets. (For details on pet poisoning, see page 265.) Antifreeze can be especially dangerous if you've transferred it from the original container into a glass jar, bottle, or other container because it doesn't look like a dangerous chemical, especially to a child. It is not uncommon for children or even adults to misidentify antifreeze in these containers as a palatable drink, consume the contents, and be poisoned.

SYMPTOMS OF POISONING

Someone who has drunk radiator antifreeze containing ethylene glycol may appear to be intoxicated. Ethylene glycol is absorbed within 30 minutes, rapidly causing symptoms. Larger doses can cause vomiting, depressed breathing, and coma within an hour. This may be followed by kidney failure within one to two days.

WHAT TO DO

Antifreeze poisoning is a clear-cut emergency. You should immediately call the regional Poison Control Center (1-800-222-1222). Sometimes, if a dilute ethylene glycol product has been ingested, calculations done by the poison center staff may determine that the child may safely remain at home.

If someone gets antifreeze in the eye but has not swallowed any of the liquid, you should rinse the eye with warm running water for 15 to 20 minutes and then call the Poison Control Center.

AT THE HOSPITAL

Doctors may use ethanol or an antidote called fomepizole intravenously to block the body's breakdown of ethylene glycol into harmful metabolites. Depending on the severity of the exposure, life support and dialysis may be needed to treat antifreeze poisoning.

AUTOMATIC DISHWASHER SOAP

Automatic dishwasher soap is an extremely harsh household

CHEMICALS

cleaner that contains various alkalis. If a child gets this soap on her skin or swallows it, severe corrosive burns can result. Phosphates, chlorine, sodium carbonate, and surfactants are typical ingredients in dishwasher detergents; they are all harmful if swallowed or touched.

A child's prognosis following contact with automatic dishwasher soap depends on how rapidly the soap is diluted, but extensive damage to the mouth, throat, and stomach are possible. The ultimate outcome depends on the extent of this damage.

SYMPTOMS OF POISONING

Automatic dishwasher soap causes an immediate reaction on contact, burning whatever tissues it touches. Swallowing this product will cause severe pain in the mouth and throat, throat swelling and breathing problems, severe stomach pain, collapse, and sometimes death.

WHAT TO DO

If your child has swallowed automatic dishwasher soap, call the regional Poison Control Center (1-800-222-1222) immediately. Do not induce vomiting. You should not give anything by mouth unless directed to do so by the poison center. If you do not have immediate access to a phone, milk or water can be given if the child is able to swallow. Never force milk or water down the throat.

If the skin or eyes come into contact with automatic dishwasher soap, immediately begin to decontaminate them by rinsing the affected area with lots of water, and contact poison control for further instructions.

AT THE HOSPITAL

Depending upon the severity of the exposure, the health care team may perform an endoscopy, a procedure in which a camera is inserted down the throat to see the extent of burns to the esophagus and the stomach. Intravenous fluids and pain medications may also be given.

BLEACH

A common disinfectant and cleaner found in almost every home, household bleach is not as toxic as many other cleaning products. In fact, it is considered to be essentially nontoxic unless very large amounts are ingested or sucked into the lungs. Poison centers receive about 20,000 calls a year concerning children who have swallowed bleach. The typical incident involves a child under age 5 who drinks bleach from a cup left unattended in the laundry room. Containing approximately 5 percent sodium hypochlorite, household bleach rarely results in significant injury if swallowed.

CAUTION!

Bleach can cause serious inhalation poisoning if it's combined with ammonia during household cleaning; this produces a toxic gas that can cause lung damage if inhaled.

WHAT TO DO

Although household bleach rarely causes injury, you should still call the Poison Control Center (1-800-222-1222) if your child swallows any. In many cases, children do not need medical attention if they have no symptoms—but that should always be the poison center's decision.

A common remedy for a child who has drunk small quantities of bleach is to administer a glass of milk or water, but you should wait for the poison center or your local emergency care personnel to recommend a specific liquid.

CHEMICALS

If skin or eyes come into contact with household bleach, immediately begin to decontaminate them by rinsing with lots of water, and contact poison control for further instructions.

BUTTON BATTERIES

If accidentally swallowed, tiny button batteries used in watches, calculators, cameras, and hearing aids usually pass through a child's digestive tract without any problem. However, these small batteries may cause internal burns if they become lodged in the esophagus.

 WHAT TO DO

If your child has swallowed a miniature battery, you should contact your regional Poison Control Center (1-800-222-1222), your physician, or the National Button Battery Ingestion hotline at 202-625-3333 (collect calls accepted). Expect to be directed to go to a health care facility where an X-ray can be performed to see where the button battery is located. If the battery is lodged in the esophagus, it will have to be removed. If it is in the stomach or further along in the digestive tract, it will be allowed to pass over the ensuing days.

CARBON MONOXIDE

Carbon monoxide (CO) kills more Americans than any other poison. Nearly 5,000 people are treated each year in hospitals for poisoning by this colorless, odorless, deadly gas. Carbon monoxide is produced when fuel is burned—in cars, lawn mowers, furnaces, hot water heaters, oil burners, kerosene heaters, fireplaces, and grills.

Breathing CO prevents the body's red blood cells from carrying oxygen, essentially starving vital organs. Because children are so much smaller than adults, it doesn't take much carbon monoxide gas to cause harm.

Most fuel-powered devices are designed or installed in such a way as to reduce the risk of CO poisoning, but they can malfunction or be used improperly. For example, a blocked chimney flue or a portable generator left running in an enclosed space can cause CO gas to rise to deadly levels.

Recovery from significant carbon monoxide poisoning may be slow. Depending on the exposure level, the length of exposure, and the pre-existing health condition of the person exposed, permanent brain damage can develop. Those who lose consciousness are at the most risk for permanent damage.

SYMPTOMS OF POISONING

The symptoms of carbon monoxide poisoning are insidious and mimic many other diseases, such as the flu. The first symptoms often appear as dizziness, headache, weakness, fatigue, sleepiness, nausea and vomiting, confusion, shortness of breath, fainting, and disorientation. As the level of the gas rises in the blood, the person exposed becomes more confused, and may lose consciousness, stop breathing, and die.

CO is particularly dangerous because the cause of the symptoms is often not recognized by either those exposed or by health care providers. Babies and young children are at particularly high risk, but so are the elderly and anyone with anemia or a history of heart disease.

WHAT TO DO

If you suspect carbon monoxide poisoning, get the child out into fresh air immediately. Call 911 right away if any symptoms are evident; if available, oxygen should be administered immediately in such a situation. Artificial respiration may need to be given if the child has stopped breathing, until emergency help arrives.

CHEMICALS

AT THE HOSPITAL

Doctors will administer oxygen, monitor vital signs, and take blood tests. In certain cases, hyperbaric oxygen may be administered.

PREVENTION!

Install a carbon monoxide detector on each floor of your home, and an additional detector near any major gas-burning appliances (such as a furnace or a water heater). Detectors that meet the UL (Underwriters Laboratories) standards measure both high CO concentrations over short periods and low concentrations over long periods. Detectors should sound an alarm before the level of gas becomes dangerous. Inexpensive cardboard or plastic detectors that change color (but don't sound an alarm) aren't particularly useful, since you have to be looking at them to realize there's a problem.

If you've got only one carbon monoxide detector, the Consumer Product Safety Commission recommends that you install it near the bedrooms so the alarm will be sure to wake you if you're sleeping. But if possible, add detectors on every level in your house, and in every bedroom.

When you're installing detectors, remember not to install them directly above or beside furnaces and other fuel-burning devices, since these may normally release an inconsequential bit of carbon monoxide when they kick on. Likewise, you shouldn't put a detector within 15 feet of cooking appliances, or near humid areas such as bathrooms. Keep in mind that if carbon monoxide is coming from combustion appliances such as home heaters, it will rise with the warmer air. For this reason, experts suggest that you place your detectors on the ceiling.

Have a qualified service technician routinely inspect your central and room heating appliances (including water heaters and gas dryers) each year. Any area where you're using an unvented gas or kerosene space heater must be well ventilated, and doors leading to other rooms should be opened for maximum ventilation.

WHAT TO DO IF THE ALARM SOUNDS

If your carbon monoxide detector's alarm goes off, turn off your appliances and any other source of combustion right away, and immediately open all your doors and windows to bring in fresh air. You'll need to call a qualified technician to have the problem checked and fixed before you restart your appliances. If anyone in the house is experiencing symptoms of carbon monoxide poisoning (headaches, dizziness, vomiting), call the fire department and immediately move everyone out into the fresh air. Do not reenter the premises for any reason until the problem has been corrected.

To figure out where the carbon monoxide is coming from, have a professional check:

Gas or oil furnaces

The concentrations of carbon monoxide in flue gases should be measured, and all connections to flue pipes and venting systems checked for cracks, gaps, rust, corrosion, or gunk. The professional also should check the filters for dirt or blockages, and the combustion chamber and heat exchanger for cracks, holes, metal fatigue, or corrosion. Furnace flame, burners, and ignition systems also should be checked. If a natural gas furnace has a mostly yellow, flat flame, it is not burning efficiently, and probably releasing higher-than-normal levels of carbon monoxide. Oil furnaces with a similar problem have an oily odor.

Heating-unit venting systems and chimneys

Look for debris, animal nests, cracks, holes, or cave-ins. A blocked chimney or venting system can force dangerous gases from the furnace back into your home.

Venting and fan systems on all fuel-burning appliances

This includes gas water heaters, clothes dryers, space heaters, and wood-burning stoves that, if not properly installed, vent carbon monoxide in rather than out.

CHEMICALS

Fireplaces

A blocked or bent fireplace chimney or flue, soot and debris, or holes could be allowing carbon monoxide exhaust back into your home.

Stove pilot lights

These can cause carbon monoxide build-up if they aren't vented to the outside. Fireplace pilot lights, which also produce carbon monoxide, should be checked regularly.

RECOGNIZE THE WARNING SIGNS

Carbon monoxide is odorless and invisible, but these indicators could tip you off to a possible problem and avert a tragedy:

✗ Appliances that make unusual sounds, have odd smells, or keep shutting off.

✗ Rust or stains on vents and chimneys.

✗ Household members who become sick only when at home but improve when away or in fresh air.

✗ Animals that get sick along with the humans in the home.

CAUSTICS

DRAIN CLEANERS, OVEN CLEANERS, TOILET BOWL CLEANERS

When categorizing household cleaners, you could think of caustics as the mean and nasty variety. Employed in the toughest jobs, they eat up and destroy whatever dirt stands in their way—something to think about if there are young children in the vicinity.

Some of the most dangerous cleaning ingredients are the sodium hydroxide and lye found in products formulated to unclog drains or clean ovens. (Fortunately, oven cleaners are now much less common due to the popularity of self-cleaning ovens.) You'll need to be especially vigilant with busy toddlers, who are most likely to get into these products that are so often stored under a sink.

These corrosive cleaners can eat right through the skin, and if swallowed can burn the mouth, esophagus, and stomach. The extent of injury depends on how much drain or oven cleaner the child has consumed, and the eventual outcome hinges on how much damage there was to the child's mouth, throat, and digestive system.

SYMPTOMS OF POISONING

Drain, oven, and toilet bowl cleaners can cause severe pain in the mouth and throat, breathing problems due to a swollen throat, severe stomach pain, diarrhea and vomiting, a rapid drop in blood pressure, and shock and death. Following the initial burns, the exposed child may later develop perforation of the digestive tract as the damaged tissue becomes softened. With healing, the digestive tract may become scarred, making it difficult for food to pass through narrowed areas. Those with extensive damage to the esophagus are at high risk for the later development (decades later) of esophageal cancer.

WHAT TO DO

Ingestion of drain or oven cleaner constitutes a medical emergency; call the regional Poison Control Center (1-800-222-1222) or dial 911 immediately. Do not induce vomiting and do not try to neutralize the cleaner with vinegar or lemon juice—this may cause more severe burning. Before giving anything by mouth, you should check with the poison center.

CHEMICALS

If you do not have immediate access to a telephone, give water or milk immediately if the child is able to fully swallow, does not have difficulty breathing, and is completely awake.

If the skin or eyes have come into contact with drain cleaner, immediately begin to rinse with lots of water and contact the Poison Control Center for further instructions.

AT THE HOSPITAL

Depending upon the severity of the exposure, the health care team may perform an endoscopy, a procedures in which a camera is inserted into the throat to see the extent of burns to the esophagus and stomach. Intravenous fluids and pain medications may also be given. For inhalation, oxygen may be given.

DUPLICATING FLUID   SEE METHANOL

FURNITURE POLISH   SEE HYDROCARBONS

GASOLINE   SEE HYDROCARBONS

HYDROCARBONS

This broad category of poisons includes substances such as gasoline, kerosene, benzene, formaldehyde, lamp oil, lighter fluid, motor oil, paint thinners, and furniture polish.

With so many of these products stored in houses and garages, it's little wonder hydrocarbons are among the leading causes of poisoning death in children. Many youngsters under the age of five, for example, are poisoned by swallowing gasoline, kerosene, or paint thinner, but most recover.

At greater risk are teenagers who intentionally breathe the fumes of these products to become intoxicated. This type of drug abuse is called huffing (when a cloth saturated with the hydrocarbon is held over the nose and mouth), sniffing (when the chemical is held directly to the nose or placed inside it), or bagging (when the hydrocarbon is placed in a bag and the opening then placed around the nose and mouth). No matter what the variation, the umbrella term for these dangerous practices is volatile substance abuse.

SYMPTOMS OF POISONING

These substances may cause irritation and/or burns in the mouth and throat, difficulty breathing, stomach pain, diarrhea, vomiting, a drop in blood pressure, and collapse. A child commonly will cough and/or choke after swallowing a hydrocarbon. A burning sensation can develop in the stomach, and vomiting may ensue. Hydrocarbon ingestion also may cause drowsiness, poor coordination, confusion, coma, and seizures.

If the lungs are significantly affected, the victim continues to cough intensely, breathing becomes rapid, and the skin may become bluish because of low levels of oxygen in the blood.

Inhaling hydrocarbons, especially after exertion or stress, may induce fatal heartbeat irregularities. Swallowed hydrocarbons also can enter and irritate the lungs, a serious condition in itself (chemical pneumonitis), and can lead to severe pneumonia. Lung involvement is a particular problem with thin, easy-flowing (low viscosity and high volatility) hydrocarbons such as lamp oils.

WHAT TO DO

In the event of suspected hydrocarbon poisoning, call the regional Poison Control Center immediately (1-800-222-1222). Wash affected skin and remove any contaminated clothing. If the child has stopped coughing and choking and if not much of the sub-

CHEMICALS

stance was swallowed, treatment at home may be possible, but only under the guidance of the poison center. If there are any significant breathing problems, you should dial 911 immediately. People who inhale hydrocarbons into their lungs can deteriorate in less than an hour and require life support.

AT THE HOSPITAL

If your child is having breathing problems, hospitalization is essential. If pneumonia or chemical pneumonitis develops, hospital treatment can include oxygen or, in severe cases, a breathing machine. Recovery time after this type of poisoning can range from a day to months. In the worst cases, permanent lung damage can result. Brain damage may occur in those who collapse if CPR or other resuscitation efforts are delayed.

KEROSENE   SEE HYDROCARBONS

METHANOL

Also known as methyl alcohol or wood alcohol, methanol is contained in windshield washing fluid, de-icers, duplicating fluid, antifreeze, shellac, perfumes, solvents, and paint removers. Many of these products are typically stored in garages and sheds, where inquisitive toddlers may find and drink them.

Much more poisonous than the ethyl alcohol in a cocktail, methanol takes much longer to be eliminated from the body and can cause blindness and death. A liquid at room temperature, methanol evaporates quickly. It can be swallowed, inhaled as a vapor, or absorbed through the skin.

SYMPTOMS OF POISONING

Because methanol is metabolized so slowly, it may take anywhere from hours to days before symptoms appear. In the first hours after drinking this solution, the child may seem to be drunk, but once methanol is transformed into formaldehyde in the body, it can trigger dizziness, fatigue, headache, nausea and vomiting, severe stomach pain, or vision problems.

In larger doses, symptoms may progress to shallow breathing, bluish skin, a rapid drop in blood pressure, coma, and eventually death from respiratory arrest. Organ damage can occur; the eyes are especially at risk.

Breathing methanol fumes can cause dizziness, eye irritation, nausea, and visual problems. Inhaling extremely large amounts of the fumes can be fatal.

WHAT TO DO

If you believe your child may have come into contact with methanol, call the regional Poison Control Center (1-800-222-1222) immediately. The staff at the poison center will determine if the exposure was serious enough to warrant a visit to the hospital.

AT THE HOSPITAL

Doctors may use ethanol or an antidote called fomepizole intravenously to block the body's breakdown of methanol into harmful metabolites. Folic acid or leucovorin in high doses may be administered to help rid the body of any harmful metabolites that may have been formed. Depending on the severity of the exposure, life support and dialysis may be needed to treat methanol poisoning.

MOUTHWASH

While not inherently poisonous, many mouthwashes contain up

CHEMICALS

to 20 percent alcohol, which can be harmful to children if they swallow it. In just one year, 34 life-threatening cases of pediatric mouthwash poisoning and one death were reported in the United States. Because many of these products have sweet tastes and pretty colors, they may be especially attractive to young children. Mouthwash containing alcohol should never be given to children under age six.

SYMPTOMS OF POISONING

As with alcohol, small amounts of mouthwash can lead to a drop in your child's blood sugar, and cause intoxication or seizures.

WHAT TO DO

If you suspect a child under age six has swallowed mouthwash containing alcohol, call the regional Poison Control Center (1-800-222-1222) immediately. The staff at the poison center will determine if the exposure was serious enough to warrant a visit to the hospital.

PREVENTION!

To avoid the risk of having your child drink alcohol-containing mouthwash, buy and use only alcohol-free brands.

PAINT (OIL-BASED)

Curious toddlers may occasionally swallow some oil-based paint, which can be toxic because of the hydrocarbons contained in these products. Some artist's paints also have heavy metals such as lead, mercury, cobalt, and barium added as pigment. These heavy metals can cause additional toxicity if consumed in sufficient quantities.

SYMPTOMS OF POISONING

Paint ingestions rarely cause symptoms. But swallowing prob-

CHEMICALS

lems, stomach pain, nausea and vomiting, diarrhea, dizziness, depression, rapid heartbeat, nervousness, confusion, stupor, and loss of consciousness have been reported.

WHAT TO DO

Call the regional Poison Control Center (1-800-222-1222). Do not induce vomiting. If the child is conscious, you can give a small amount of milk or water to stop any irritation or burning of the mouth and throat.

AT THE HOSPITAL

If the child is continuously vomiting, an intravenous line may be placed, and fluids may be given. Blood tests may be done.

PAINT THINNER   SEE HYDROCARBONS

PERFUMES   SEE METHANOL

CHEMICALS

PESTICIDES

Pesticides are a major cause of poisoning because of the multitude of potential sources of exposure. In fact, the term "pesticide" is applied to a broad range of different chemicals, with targets ranging from weeds to rats. According to the American Association of Poison Control Centers, there were 46,929 pediatric pesticide exposures and two fatalities reported in one recent year. A survey by the U.S. Environmental Protection Agency found that 47 percent of all households with children had at least one pesticide stored in an unlocked cabinet within 4 feet of the ground.

Child-resistant packaging and the development of safer

products, like pyrethroids, have helped to decrease the number and severity of poisonings from pesticides. The most commonly used pesticides today include carbamates, organophosphates, pyrethroids, and, to a decreasing extent, organochlorines.

ORGANOCHLORINES

Organochlorines such as DDT, chlordane, aldrin, endrin, dieldrin, and kepone are highly effective insecticides. However, their use in North America has significantly decreased over the past decades because of environmental concerns, and they are no longer sold to the general public.

Lindane, an organochlorine used to treat conditions such as scabies and lice, is still available by prescription and may be found in the home. In California, however, it is considered to be a carcinogen and its use has been banned. The U.S. Food and Drug Administration in 1995 labeled lindane a "second-line treatment" for lice because the agency believes there are safer alternatives that should be used first, especially in young children.

SYMPTOMS OF POISONING

Typical symptoms after ingestion include only nausea, vomiting, and stomach pain. Seizures may occur rarely.

WHAT TO DO

Remove the exposed child from the exposure source, strip off any contaminated clothing, and cleanse the skin with soap and water. Call the regional Poison Control Center number (1-800-222-1222) immediately. The staff at the poison center will determine if the exposure was serious enough to warrant a visit to the hospital.

AT THE HOSPITAL

Depending on the severity of the exposure and the type of organochlorine agent, an intravenous line may be inserted and blood may be drawn for tests. If seizures develop, benzodiazepines will be given.

ORGANOPHOSPHATES AND CARBAMATES

Many different organophosphate and carbamate products are used as insecticides. The organophosphate category includes parathion, chlorpyrifos, diazinon, fenthion, and malathion. Carbamates include aldicarb, carbaryl, carbofuran, dioxacarb, and etrofolan.

SYMPTOMS OF POISONING

Poisoning from these chemicals may cause nausea, vomiting, diarrhea, constricted pupils, involuntary urination, wheezing, breathing problems, uncontrollable tearing, increased saliva production, excessive sweating, confusion, agitation, seizures, and coma, along with weakness and paralysis.

WHAT TO DO

Get the exposed child away from the source of the insecticide, remove contaminated clothing, and cleanse the skin with soap and water. Call the regional Poison Control Center number (1-800-222-1222) immediately. The staff at the poison center will determine if the exposure was serious enough to warrant a visit to the hospital.

AT THE HOSPITAL

Depending on the severity of the exposure and the type of chemical, an intravenous line may be inserted and blood may be drawn for tests. Atropine is an antidote used for both organophosphate and carbamate poisoning that may be given to patients with symptoms. Pralidoxime chloride is an antidote used primarily for organophosphate poisoning, and may be administered if necessary. If seizures develop, a benzodiazepine (an anti-anxiety drug) will be given. In the rare cases in which life-threatening symptoms develop, life support may be required.

CHEMICALS

PYRETHRINS AND SYNTHETIC PYRETHROIDS

Pyrethrins are natural insecticides derived from the chrysanthemum plant. These products are much less toxic to people than to insects because the human liver quickly metabolizes them. They kill by interfering with the insect's nervous system. Pyrethroids are the synthetic form of pyrethrins.

SYMPTOMS OF POISONING

These substances may cause allergic reactions, especially in children allergic to ragweed pollen. Symptoms include eye irritation, wheezing, cough, nose drainage, and itching. Rarely, seizures may occur if these products are swallowed.

WHAT TO DO

Remove the exposed child from the source of the contamination, take off any contaminated clothing, and cleanse the skin with soap and water. Call the regional Poison Control Center hotline (1-800-222-1222) immediately. The staff at the poison center will determine if the exposure was serious enough to warrant a visit to the hospital.

AT THE HOSPITAL

Allergic reactions may be treated with diphenhydramine, albuterol, steroids, and epinephrine, depending on the severity of symptoms. Seizures may be treated with a benzodiazepine.

RAT POISONS (ALUMINUM, ZINC PHOSPHIDE)

Aluminum phosphide and zinc phosphide are rat poisons. They are also commonly used to eradicate moles. These products are often sold in pellet form, and react with water to produce phosphine gas. If highly concentrated phosphine gas is accidentally inhaled, it can cause widespread death to cells.

SYMPTOMS OF POISONING

If pellets are ingested, abdominal pain, nausea, and vomiting may develop. Exposure to formed phosphine gas may cause eye irritation, throat discomfort, cough, and shortness of breath. Symptoms may be delayed until several days after exposure.

WHAT TO DO

Remove the child from the source of exposure, remove contaminated clothing, and cleanse the skin with soap and water. Call the regional Poison Control Center (1-800-222-1222) immediately. The staff at the poison center will determine if the exposure was serious enough to warrant a trip to the hospital.

AT THE HOSPITAL

No antidote exists for aluminum phosphide or zinc phosphide poisoning, so treatment is limited to easing symptoms.

WEED KILLER (PARAQUAT AND DIQUAT)

Paraquat and diquat are effective weed killers that were once commonly found in stores, although they are now used less often in the United States.

SYMPTOMS OF POISONING

Paraquat and diquat have caustic properties. Initially, if a child drinks either of these herbicides, the chemical may cause irritation of the mouth, throat discomfort, breathing problems, abdominal pain, nausea, and vomiting. Paraquat may cause delayed lung damage, and both products may cause delayed kidney damage. Those who survive the lung injury induced by paraquat may develop a condition called pulmonary fibrosis, which can cause chronic shortness of breath.

WHAT TO DO

Get the exposed person away from the chemical, remove any

clothing that may have been contaminated, and cleanse the skin with soap and water. Call the regional Poison Control Center number (1-800-222-1222) immediately. The staff at the poison center will determine if the exposure was serious enough to warrant a visit to the hospital.

AT THE HOSPITAL

No antidote exists for these products. Intravenous fluids and pain medications may be given. Depending upon the severity of the exposure, doctors may perform an endoscopy, a procedure in which a camera is put down the throat to see the extent of burns to the esophagus and the stomach. A patient with severe breathing problems will be given oxygen. Worst cases can lead to lung or kidney damage.

PLAYGROUND EQUIPMENT
(PRESSURE-TREATED WOOD)

Between 1930 and 2004, wooden playground sets and outdoor decks were built with lumber treated with chromated copper arsenate (CCA), a registered chemical pesticide used to preserve wood from rotting. CCA contains arsenic, chromium, and copper. Beginning in the 1970s, in fact, most of the wood used to build outdoor residential settings has been CCA-treated wood. In 2002, however, the U.S. Environmental Protection Agency reached an agreement with manufacturers of wood preservative products containing CCA to cancel the preservative's registration for use in virtually all residential applications. As of December 31, 2003, it is illegal to treat lumber for residential use with CCA. However, many structures built before the ban are found throughout this country in backyards and playgrounds.

The U.S. Consumer Product Safety Commission has been concerned about CCA-treated wood in playground equipment because exposure to arsenic might increase a child's risk of developing lung or bladder cancer over a lifetime. Specifically, children can be exposed to the arsenic by playing on playsets or touching toys made from CCA-treated wood and then putting their hands into their mouths.

Because arsenic is a known carcinogen, some consumer advocates want to see a more vigorous regulatory approach to the problem. But the EPA has stated it does not believe there is any reason to remove or replace existing CCA-treated structures, including decks and playground equipment.

PREVENTION!

To minimize the risk from arsenic in CCA-treated playsets, you should thoroughly wash your child's hands with soap and water immediately after outdoor play on such equipment and especially before eating. Children also should be discouraged from snacking while playing on CCA-treated playgrounds.

If you are planning to build a playset or deck at your home, there are a number of non-arsenic-containing preservatives registered by the EPA to pressure treat wood. Ammonium copper quaternary (ACQ) and copper boron azole (CBA) are common ones. Ask for ACQ- or CBA-treated wood at your lumberyard or home improvement store.

Keep in mind that pre-assembled playground equipment made of other non-arsenic-containing components is also available— including woods such as cedar and redwood, and non-wood alternatives such as metal and plastic.

If you have an existing CCA-treated structure, available data suggest that applying a coating to the wood at least once a year can reduce the leaching of arsenic. Oil- or water-based stains that can penetrate wood surfaces are preferable to products such as paint.

SYMPTOMS OF POISONING

Exposure to CCA-treated wood does not produce any symptoms but only shows up later in life as lung or bladder cancer.

CHEMICALS

DON'T BURN PRESSURE-TREATED WOOD

Never burn pressure-treated wood in an open fire, stove, fireplace, or residential boiler. Instead, contact the U.S. Environmental Protection Agency at www.epa.gov, or call your state or local solid waste management office for instructions on how to dispose of CCA-treated wood.

RADON

CHEMICALS

Created by the decay of naturally occurring radium and uranium in rocks and soil, this invisible and odorless radioactive gas can seep into the basement of a house. Once indoors, it breaks down into harmful elements that can attach to dust particles and damage the lungs when inhaled. One in 15 American homes throughout the United States has radon levels high enough to pose a health risk, according to the U.S. Environmental Protection Agency. Indeed, more than 20,000 Americans die of radon-related lung cancer each year, according to the U.S. Surgeon General. Worldwide, radon is responsible for 15 percent of all lung cancers.

FOR STATE-SPECIFIC INFORMATION

Radon levels can vary according to a region's geology. To find out where to get specific information about radon in your state, visit the U.S. Environmental Protection Agency's Web site at: www.epa.gov

Outdoor radon levels in the United States range from 0.02 to 0.75 pCi/L (picoCuries per liter). Most buildings draw in concentrated radon gas from the ground, but because radon is eight times heavier than air, high radon levels tend to build up only in basements and on lower floors. Congress has set the "target radon level" for homes as no higher than the average natural level outdoors—0.4 pCi/L. But about two-thirds of homes exceed that. In fact, the average radon level in U.S. homes is 1.25 pCi/L, or three times higher than the average outdoor level.

Few techniques exist to eliminate radon and their cost to homeowners is high—averaging $1,200, but running as high as $2,500. As a result, the EPA has issued only two recommendations: a 4 pCi/L "action" limit (fix your home) and a 2 pCi/L "consider action" limit (*consider* fixing your home). Nearly eight million U.S. homes have radon levels above the "action limit," and nearly one out of six exceed the "consider action" limit. You should always try to reduce radon to a practical minimum. Although the 4 pCi/L level has become an acceptable benchmark for real estate transactions, it still carries risks equivalent to smoking 10 cigarettes a day, according to the EPA.

CHEMICALS

PREVENTION!

You can obtain sensors (typically placed in the basement) that detect radon. If you do discover excessive radon, you can purchase equipment that can vent radon from the basement. Basements with access to the outdoors and daylight can be vented daily via windows and doors.

If you want to find a qualified radon service professional to test or treat your home, or you want to purchase a do-it-yourself radon measurement device, contact personnel at your state radon organization, which also can advise you of any state-specific radon measurement or mitigation requirements.

Alternatively, you can contact one or both of the two privately run radon proficiency programs that offer proficiency listing, accreditation, and certification of radon technicians. (For contact information, see page 297.)

SYMPTOMS OF POISONING

There are no symptoms of acute radon contamination other than the eventual development of lung cancer. Typically, cancer may occur from five to 25 years after exposure. There is no evidence that other respiratory diseases (such as asthma) are caused by radon exposure, and there's no evidence that children are at any greater risk of radon-induced lung cancer than adults.

SWIMMING POOL CLEANERS

Ingesting a variety of products used to clean and keep home swimming pools germ-free may cause poisoning. Often stored in sheds or garages, such products should always be locked up and kept away from children. These pool cleaners include mild acids in liquid form, as well as chlorine in tablet, granule, and liquid form. Chlorine products also carry the risk of inhalation poisoning by chlorine dust or fumes formed when chlorine is mixed with other chemicals.

SYMPTOMS OF POISONING

Swimming pool acids may burn the skin. They also can cause breathing problems if inhaled, or severe stomach pain, nausea, and bloody vomiting if ingested. A child who eats chlorine tablets or inhales chlorine dust may experience breathing problems, throat swelling, severe pain in the throat, severe pain or burning in the nose, eyes, and ears, or on the lips or tongue. Other symptoms can include vision loss, severe stomach pain, vomiting, burns of the esophagus, blood in the stool, low blood pressure, and collapse.

CHEMICALS

WHAT TO DO

If your child has swallowed any of these pool products, consider it a potential medical emergency and call the regional Poison Control Center (1-800-222-1222) immediately. Do not induce vomiting. Do not give anything by mouth unless directed to do so by the poison center. If you do not have immediate access to a phone, you can give your child milk or water if she is able to swallow. However, never force milk or water down a child's throat. If the skin or eyes come into contact with these products, immediately begin to decontaminate by rinsing with lots of water, and contact the poison center for further instructions.

AT THE HOSPITAL

Depending upon the severity of the exposure, doctors may place an endoscopy, a tiny camera down the throat, to see the extent of burns to the esophagus and stomach. Intravenous fluids and pain medications also may be given. Oxygen and albuterol, a bronchodilator, may be given if acids were inhaled.

TOILET BOWL CLEANERS   SEE CAUSTICS

WINDSHIELD WASHER SOLUTION
SEE METHANOL

CHEMICALS

7

BE CAREFUL IN THERE

TOXIC WATER CREATURES

While there are some quite deadly poisonous sea dwellers in other parts of the world, the most common toxic creature that people might contact in North American waters is the jellyfish. These oddly formed invertebrates wash up on sandy beaches all along the eastern and western coasts. Occasionally kids and adults alike may come in contact with other poisonous or venomous creatures found in the water—including sting rays, sea anemones, water snakes, and sea urchins.

CATFISH

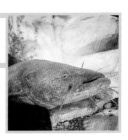

Catfish (also known as bullheads) are ugly but tasty bottom-dwelling fish with cat-like whiskers around the mouth. They are typically found in muddy rivers and lakes, and in tropical, subtropical, and temperate waters throughout the world; species of catfish can be found on every continent except Antarctica. All catfish have sharp barbs on their fins that inject poison when they jab an enemy. Remember, it's their fin barbs that sting, not their whiskers. Youngsters who are stung by catfish are usually fishing or swimming at the time. In many cases, they simply step on an unwary fish.

SYMPTOMS OF POISONING

Pain and inflammation occur at the site where a catfish has stung; an infection may develop at that spot later. Portions of the stinging apparatus may become embedded in the skin, causing continued discomfort.

WHAT TO DO

To relieve pain from a sting, immerse the affected area in water that is as hot as possible without being scalding. Remove embedded spines with tweezers, and scrub and irrigate the wound with fresh water. The wound should not be taped or sewn together. To help relieve pain, take one or two acetaminophen (Tylenol) tablets every four hours or one or two ibuprofen (Motrin, Advil) tablets every six to eight hours.

AT THE DOCTOR'S OFFICE

Oral antibiotics are usually prescribed for stings that become infected.

JELLYFISH

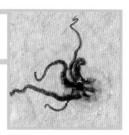

Although the sting of some jellyfish can be quite toxic and even deadly, the sting of many found in the waters off North America is harmless to humans. True jellyfish include about 200 species, only about 70 of which can really hurt you. Typically found drifting along the shoreline, all jellyfish have four, eight, or more dangling tentacles that sting when they are touched. The more dangerous jellies that might be encountered by bathers include:

Lion's mane, found in the Atlantic Ocean from above the Arctic Circle to Florida; in the Gulf of Mexico; and in the Pacific from Alaska to southern California.

Portuguese man-of-war, found in the Gulf of Mexico.

Sea nettle, found in the Chesapeake Bay, in the Pacific from Alaska to southern California, in the Atlantic from Massachusetts to Florida, and in the Gulf of Mexico.

Relatives of corals and sea anemones, these invertebrates have no head, brain, heart, eyes, or bones. Jellyfish stings most commonly occur in tropical or warm waters, when the creatures' trailing tentacles contact a bather's skin. They cause a significant number of injuries along coastal areas in the United States. Jellies are also dangerous after storms have broken them and flung them across the beach, where—although dead and dry— they can still sting an unsuspecting person who touches one or tries to pick one up.

Jellyfish, which swim along the surface, come in lots of different sizes and shapes, but they are all often almost transparent. Because some types have very long tentacles, it's also possible to be stung without ever seeing the top of the jellyfish floating on the surface of the water.

PREVENTION!

At the beach, always check for jellyfish warning signs before entering the water. If you see a jelly or part of one that has been washed up on the sand, remember that it can still cause a sting if handled or stepped on; make sure you and your children stay well clear of it.

SYMPTOMS OF POISONING

Severe, burning pain and a red welt on the skin are the typical symptoms of a jellyfish sting. Some people also experience headache, nausea and vomiting, muscle cramps, diarrhea, convulsions, and breathing problems.

The sting of a Portuguese man-of-war jellyfish is especially potent, although rarely fatal. It can cause hives, numbness, and severe chest, abdominal, and limb pain.

If a swimmer is stung while in the water, the sudden pain may cause him to jerk away, which stimulates the tentacles to release even more poison. On shore, additional toxin is released if the victim tries to rip off the sticky threads.

WHAT TO DO

If you are your child are attacked, it is not important to identify the type of jellyfish. If the swimmer is stung at a guarded beach, check with the lifeguards on duty. They can render minor first aid or, for more serious cases, call for emergency medical evacuation assistance.

Decontamination should be started immediately. If specific decontaminating agents aren't readily available, the skin can be rinsed with sea water or saline solution to remove the remnants of the jellyfish, or you can liberally apply vinegar, baking soda, or a solution of dilute (one-quarter strength) household ammonia to the affected area.

Do not apply isopropyl alcohol. It can trigger further discharge of the poison into the system, and isn't recommended as a decontaminant.

Vinegar and ammonia compresses may be applied continuously. A paste made from unseasoned meat tenderizer or the fruit of the papaya also has been reported to significantly relieve the pain associated with jellyfish stings. Calamine lotion may help ease the burning sensation, and over-the-counter painkillers also may help. If meat tenderizer is used, it should be applied for no longer than 15 minutes (especially if the victim is a child). The other decontaminants mentioned above should be applied until the pain of the sting is relieved, or for up to 30 minutes for the greatest benefit.

Following decontamination, any remaining tentacles should be removed. You can do this by covering the area with shaving cream or a paste made of baking soda and water, and then using a razor to scrape off the tentacles. At the scene, you can cover the area with a paste made of sand and sea water, then scrape the affected skin with a shell or a plastic credit card. After removing the remaining tentacles, a decontaminant should be reapplied for an additional 15 minutes.

Jellyfish stings may cause an allergic reaction; mild reactions can be treated with Benadryl.

AT THE HOSPITAL

A severe allergic reaction to a jellyfish sting is a medical emergency and requires a visit to the emergency room.

WATER CREATURES

SEA ANEMONES

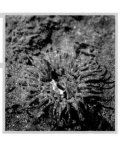

These common sea creatures may look like flowers, but they're actually predatory animals. There are thousands of varieties, ranging from a few inches to one-and-a-half feet long, all quite different from each other but sharing at least one trait: the ability to sting. Sea anemones, like their close relatives jellyfish and corals, bear tentacles lined with stinging cells. A sting is not typically fatal by itself, but if it causes shock, it could lead to drowning.

The larval forms of some anemones can find their way under kids' bathing suits. Then when the stinging cells discharge, a child may feel a tingling sensation while in the water. Itching and burning become more pronounced if a freshwater shower is taken while still wearing the suit. A red, raised rash develops in the affected areas, along with intense itching or pain. This condition is referred to as *sea bather's eruption*. Severe toxic reactions may include headache, fever, chills, and vomiting.

SYMPTOMS OF POISONING

Effects of the sting from a sea anemone are usually localized, causing burning, itching, swelling, and redness. Eventually, the skin sloughs off. This may be followed by multiple abscesses. More general symptoms include fever, chills, abdominal pain, nausea and vomiting, diarrhea, headache, and thirst.

WHAT TO DO

Soak the affected area in water that's as hot as possible without being scalding, for up to one hour, or while on the way to the doctor. A paste of baking soda and water, or calamine lotion, can be applied to the sting to relieve pain. The ulcers caused by a sea anemone are usually slow to heal.

AT THE DOCTOR'S OFFICE

Oral antibiotics are usually prescribed for stings that become infected.

SEA URCHINS

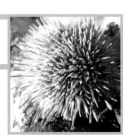

Sea urchins are typically found in warm water around rocks or shipwrecks, where they will sting swimmers or divers even through shoes and gloves. These round sea creatures are about the size of a tennis ball, with sharp, radiating spines. Of all the sea urchins, the long-spined variety (*Diadema setosum*) causes the most injuries. Red sea urchins are less venomous but still troublesome; in addition to their poison-tipped spines, they have nasty three-pronged biting teeth.

SYMPTOMS OF POISONING

The sting of a sea urchin is rarely fatal but can be quite painful, causing a throbbing sensation that may remain localized at the wound site or spread throughout the body, lasting for several hours. The affected area may become red, swollen, or numb; this may be followed by muscle weakness. A purple stain around the wound is simply caused by a pigment in the spine, and is not in itself dangerous.

WHAT TO DO

Contact medical help immediately, either by calling the Poison Control Center (1-800-222-1222) or your physician. The wound should be flushed with either salt or fresh water; the affected area should then be soaked in hot water, to help deactivate the poison. Heat should continue to be applied for 30 minutes to an hour.

WATER CREATURES

AT THE HOSPITAL

Embedded spines should be removed; but if they break off, surgery may be needed to get them out.

STINGRAYS

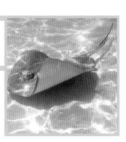

The stingray is one of the most common causes of marine venom poisonings in the United States; about 2,000 stings are reported each year. Stingrays prefer shallow, warm coastal waters along sandy beaches. Some ray species are found in fresh water, some in salt, and others can survive in both. The Atlantic stingray can be found on the eastern coast of North and Central America, and as far north as the Chesapeake Bay during the warm months of summer and early autumn. As the temperature drops, they migrate south.

Stingrays are generally peaceful bottom dwellers. Most incidents occur when a swimmer accidentally steps on a ray buried in the sand. When that happens, the stingray hurls its barbed tail up in defense, striking the person's foot or leg. Hands and arms also can be injured when trying to remove a hook from a stingray caught while fishing.

The stinging apparatus of this ray consists of one or more barbs and two venom-containing grooves; a venom gland is located at the base of the tail. Thus, an injury from a stingray includes poisoning by venom injection as well as possibly significant lacerations and puncture wounds.

SYMPTOMS OF POISONING

Stingray venom produces immediate, excruciating pain out of proportion to what might be expected based on the wound appearance alone. The pain usually peaks in about one or two hours, then starts to subside over several hours. Potential body-wide symptoms include weakness, nausea, muscle cramps, vomiting, heart rhythm disturbances, seizures, and coma.

WHAT TO DO

The wound site should be rinsed thoroughly and then the affected area should be immersed in hot water (109-113°F) for 30 to 90 minutes. This helps destabilize some of the injected venom and provides significant pain control. Health care personnel should evaluate all puncture wounds from stingrays immediately, because these wounds are notorious for becoming infected if not treated appropriately.

AT THE HOSPITAL

Pain medications may be given, and the physician may explore and thoroughly cleanse the wound. X-ray or ultrasound imaging may be performed in an attempt to see if any remaining pieces of the stingray's barb remain in the wound. If indicated, a tetanus shot and antibiotics also may be administered.

WATER MOCCASIN
(COTTONMOUTH)

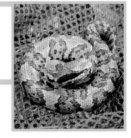

There is only one poisonous North American water snake—the water moccasin, nicknamed the "cottonmouth" because of the white color inside its mouth. This aquatic pit viper, found throughout the southeastern United States, is particularly dangerous because it won't move away if it's disturbed. In fact, sometimes it will even aggressively approach an intruder.

However, you'll still get a warning before it strikes—the cottonmouth will repeatedly open its mouth wide, showing the white interior, before biting. Powerful jaws allow this snake to latch on during a bite, so instead of the quick strike-and-release pattern of its cousin the copperhead, you'll feel a slow, dogged chomp.

Unlike other water snakes, the water moccasin swims with its head well above water, so it's easy to spot. Although sometimes seen sunning itself on a rock, this snake is most active at night, and is one of the few snakes that will feed on dead animals.

Typically more than three feet long, an adult water moccasin has a broad head and a black, olive, or brown body with dark cross bands. (Young snakes have bright, yellow-tipped tails.) Found in swamps, lakes, rivers, irrigation ditches, canals, and clear mountain streams, these snakes live from Virginia to the upper Florida Keys, and west to Illinois, Missouri, Oklahoma, and Texas.

SYMPTOMS OF POISONING

The bite of the water moccasin is potentially more venomous than that of the copperhead, and it can be fatal. Symptoms begin within 10 minutes of the bite. The venom destroys any skin, blood vessels, and muscle it contacts, and the victim can potentially develop bleeding disorders that could lead to death. The bite site may darken and ooze fluid while swelling spreads.

WHAT TO DO

If someone is bitten by a water moccasin, stay calm and avoid unnecessary first aid techniques such as a tourniquet, wound incision, suction, ice application, or electric shock that might only serve to delay essential treatment. Concentrate on getting expert help as quickly as possible. If any break in the skin has occurred (such as a puncture wound), immediate medical attention is critical. The regional Poison Control Center (1-800-222-1222) can direct you to the nearest health care facility that has antivenin, an antidote to snake venom.

AT THE HOSPITAL

Doctors will check the wound and possibly order blood tests. Painkillers will be administered as necessary. In the most severe cases, antivenin may be administered.

WATER CREATURES

8

EAT, DRINK, AND BE WARY

FOOD POISONING

As Americans, we assume we live in a country with one of the safest, most antiseptic food supplies in the entire world—but many people still experience bouts of "food poisoning" each year, whether they know it or not. While many cases of food poisoning only cause mild vomiting, diarrhea, and stomach pain, food-borne illness in the very young (as well as the very old and those with weak immune systems) can have tragic results. In fact, the Centers for Disease Control and Prevention (CDC) estimates 76 million people are diagnosed with food-borne illnesses each year in the United States, accounting for 325,000 hospitalizations and more than 5,000 deaths.

Still, there's good news on the horizon. A recent government report showed important declines in food-borne illnesses caused by common germs. As government regulations get more stringent and families better understand how to protect themselves against infection, officials hope the numbers will continue to fall.

There are more than 250 known food-borne diseases caused by bacteria, viruses, or parasites. Some symptoms are triggered by toxins from a germ, whereas others are caused by the body's reactions to an organism itself. People infected with food-borne germs may have no symptoms, or they may develop symptoms ranging from mild intestinal discomfort to bloody diarrhea and severe dehydration.

PREVENTION FIRST

The most important way to prevent your family from contracting a food-borne illness is by following correct cooking methods, which kill most bacteria, viruses, and parasites. At the same time, proper food preparation—including washing hands and keeping cutting boards and utensils clean—also can help stop the spread of infection. Anyone who is sick or who has diarrhea shouldn't prepare food for others. The foods that are most vulnerable to contamination during storage, preparation, cooking, or serving are meat, poultry, and eggs.

SHOPPING SMART

The first line of defense to prevent food-borne illness is to make sure the food you buy is clean and safe. Pay particular attention to how fresh, perishable foods are handled, packaged, and presented on store shelves.

As you shop. First choose food that won't perish quickly. Hold off on visiting the refrigerated or frozen food aisles until last, right before you check out.

The "sell by" date. As you select refrigerated or frozen foods, always check the "sell by" date to make sure it hasn't expired. A store that doesn't adhere to sell-by dates may not be so careful about keeping its refrigerators and freezers at the correct temperature, either. But be aware that even if the sell-by date is current, some stores don't keep their refrigerators cold enough, and the food can still spoil. Always check for unpleasant smells and appearance when opening any dairy product or other refrigerated item.

Check out the handler. When you're ordering food at the deli counter, be sure the clerk is wearing plastic gloves. Cheeses and raw meats should never be handled or weighed with bare hands. Don't buy any cooked items if you see that they were arranged touching raw foods in the display case.

Checkout safety. As you check out, place perishable or frozen foods from your cart all together to be bagged at once, so they'll stay colder and safer longer. If the grocery store is more than an hour from your home or if you're going to stop along the way, bring a cooler with ice in which to store perishables, and keep the food on the back seat if it's warm outside—not in the trunk.

BUYING FISH

Be choosy. At the seafood counter, check to see if the fish looks fresh; sniff it to make sure it doesn't have a strong fishy or ammonia odor. Eyes should look bright, clear, and full (not cloudy or sunken in). The flesh of filleted fish should appear moist and translucent.

Beware if fish is displayed in piles—the ones on top are at risk of getting warmer than the recommended 40°F. As bacteria on these top fish multiply, the juices may trickle down to fish underneath, spreading contamination. Displaying cooked and raw fish touching also may cause problems.

Next, check whether fish is displayed in pre-wrapped packages. Although packaging can protect from cross-contamination, it also insulates the fish from the cold. When packages are

FOOD POISONING

stacked, the ones on the top are more likely to deteriorate. If you're picking your own, choose one from the bottom of the refrigerated case, where it's coldest.

The meaning of fresh. When you shop at the fish counter, "fresh" is supposed to mean the product was never frozen or heated. "Fresh frozen" indicates the seafood was frozen when it was fresh (often within hours of harvest). If fish products were frozen and then thawed at the store, they should be labeled "previously frozen."

Lobsters, crabs, clams, and oysters are best when bought alive and cooked at home; only live mollusks with their shells tightly shut should be used. Throw out any clams or oysters whose shells are cracked.

When you've chosen your fish or seafood, the items should be packed separately or placed on top of the grocery bag. Seafood

SAFE SEAFOOD STORAGE TIMES

Should be used the same day they're bought:
Crabs (live), lobsters (live)

Should be used within 1 to 2 days:
Clams (fresh shucked), scallops, shrimp, squid

Should be used within 2 to 3 days:
Crabs (cooked), lobsters (cooked), mussels/clams (in shell)

Keeps for 3 to 4 days in airtight container:
Crabmeat, lobster

Keeps for 5 to 7 days:
Oysters (fresh shucked)

Keeps for 7 to 10 days:
Oysters (in shell)

Can be stored up to 6 months if unopened:
Crabmeat (pasteurized)

should be bought last and carried home in a cooler if you won't be able to refrigerate it for more than an hour.

Once you arrive home, you should keep your fish very cold and serve it within a day or so. Seafood should be stored in its wrapper in the coldest part of the refrigerator, as close to 32°F as possible. If the fish isn't prepackaged, wash it under cold running water and pat dry and then wrap in moisture-proof paper or plastic and store in an airtight container.

Live shellfish should be kept in a shallow container covered with a moist cloth or paper towel—not in an airtight bag, which could kill them. A few hours before steaming, you can submerge clams in cold salted water (add some cornmeal to help the clams spit out the sand they normally contain). Change the water several times to reduce the amount of grit.

IS YOUR MEAT OR POULTRY SAFE?

Look for the following signs of potential spoilage when buying meat or poultry:

✗ Frozen beef: white or bleached color

✗ Lamb: brown color

✗ Pork: darkened lean meat and discolored or rancid rind

✗ Poultry: soft, flabby flesh; purple or green color; stickiness; abnormal odor; darkening wing tips

MEAT AND POULTRY

Separate foods. Many stores provide plastic bags in the meat and poultry aisle. Always put your meat and poultry in these bags to prohibit juices from dripping on your other foods as you shop. If your store doesn't provide plastic bags, bring your own. As you check out, make sure all your fresh fruits and vegetables go in their own bags, separate from meat or poultry that could drip juice and contaminate them.

DECODE THOSE DATES

You'll probably notice a variety of dating systems on various food packages you buy. A "sell by" date indicates to store personnel how long a food can safely be displayed for sale. You should buy these products before the expiration date.

A "best if used by" date isn't a safety date—it's just a recommendation from the manufacturer advising when the product should be consumed for best flavor or quality. These dates don't really indicate how soon you need to use the product after you buy it. Even if the date passes once you get the product home, most items should still be safe and of good quality if you've handled them correctly. However, if the food looks or smells odd, you should throw it out.

Remember that no matter what the date says on the package, if you (or the store) have not handled the food correctly, germs can still grow and cause illness. You should always check perishable products for mold or off odors, even if the sell-by date hasn't passed; if the store has not kept the refrigeration units at the correct temperature, the food can spoil. Likewise, if you buy a big container of potato salad for a family picnic, transport it without refrigeration, and then leave it on a picnic table in the hot sun for hours, it won't be safe to eat no matter what the date says on the package.

SAFE STORAGE

Once you get home from the store, follow these safeguards:

✗ Unload the bags containing perishable goods first. If you intend to store meat or poultry in the refrigerator, it's best to leave it in the original package.

✗ Never store food under a sink with water, drain, or

heating pipes passing through, and always keep food off the floor and away from cleaning supplies.

✕ Store dry staple goods in their original packages or in airtight containers; any moisture that gets in can spoil the food. Canned foods can be stored for a long time at room temperature, but if the cans ever freeze, there could be safety problems. Throw them out without tasting if this occurs. If seams have rusted or burst, you must throw the cans out immediately.

REFRIGERATION BASICS

You should always keep your refrigerator set at 40°F or below; keep tabs on your appliance's cooling performance with a thermometer. Although proper cooling doesn't kill bacteria, it will keep them from multiplying. The fewer germs there are, the less likely that anyone in your family will get sick. Air should be able to circulate around refrigerated items, which should always be wrapped before being stored to guard against airborne bacteria.

FREEZER TIPS

✕ Freezer temperatures should always be kept at 0°F or below.

✕ When adding foods to the freezer that aren't yet frozen, don't stack them—the cold air needs to reach the center to chill each package fast.

✕ Freeze poultry and ground meat that won't be used in one or two days; freeze other meat if it won't be used in four or five days.

✕ Meat or poultry that's still in its original packaging and will be frozen longer than two or three months should be over-wrapped with clean plastic wrap or aluminum foil to prevent freezer burn.

✖ Meat or poultry that has been defrosted in the refrigerator may be refrozen before or after cooking, but thawing by any other method means it must be cooked before refreezing.

PREPARING FOOD SAFELY

One of the best ways to make sure your family's food stays safe is to take a few precautions as you prepare meals. The single most important way to prevent food-borne illness at this stage is to wash your hands before and after preparing food. It's fast and easy, but you'd be amazed at how many people don't do it. Hand washing drastically reduces bacteria and viruses on the skin—as long as you wash with soap for at least 30 seconds (long enough to sing "Yankee Doodle").

A good scrub with soap and water will kill about 96 percent of the germs. Liquid soap is just as good as bar soap, and studies have shown that plain soap is just as effective at killing germs as "antibacterial" soap. If you're wearing rings or artificial nails and touch raw hamburger or chicken, you must be especially careful to scrub those areas around them.

CUTTING BOARDS/UTENSILS

You also should wash cutting boards and utensils with hot, soapy water before allowing any food to touch their surfaces. An acrylic cutting board is best, since it can be washed in the dishwasher at high temperatures, which will kill any bacteria or viruses. Unlike wood, acrylic also resists pits and grooves from knives that allow germs to hide.

If you use a wooden cutting board, disinfect the board with a solution of 2 teaspoons of household bleach mixed with 1 quart of water at least once a week. Flush the board thoroughly with hot water after applying the bleach. It's a good idea to keep a separate cutting board just for meat and poultry.

Be sure to keep your can opener and blender blade free from food particles and debris. If you wash dishes by hand, don't let them soak in water for a long time. Wash them within two hours of soaking and let them air dry.

Bleach and commercial kitchen cleaning products are the best sanitizers, and they're really effective at killing bacteria. The kitchen sink, drain, and disposal are often hiding places for germs; you should sanitize these from time to time by pouring in a solution of 2 teaspoons of chlorine bleach to 1 quart of water. Although baking soda, lemon juice, and vinegar are touted for "killing germs" on kitchen surfaces, research has shown that they aren't as effective as chlorine.

DISHCLOTHS AND SPONGES

Scientists have found more bacteria on a typical kitchen sponge than on the rim of the toilet—in fact, the kitchen sponge and dishcloth are often the most germ-ridden spots in your house. On dry surfaces, bacteria can survive for only a few hours, but moist surfaces provide the perfect spot for germs to linger and multiply. The longer a sponge stays moist, the higher the bacterial count will be.

If you must use a sponge or dishcloth to clean counters, you should reserve one for the dishes, another to wipe up at the sink, and still one more for cleaning other kitchen surfaces. Even if you're putting the cloth or sponge into hot sudsy water, bacteria can survive. Ideally, you should discard sponges used for wiping dishes or countertops after one week. Alternatively, run them through the dishwasher every day or so. If you don't have a dishwasher, you can sanitize your sponges by putting moist ones into a microwave for one minute. (They may burn if heated longer.)

If you don't like sponges, you can keep a stack of white dishcloths in a drawer and use a fresh one each day; throw the used cloths in the laundry and run them through a hot wash cycle with detergent and chlorine bleach.

THAWING MEAT

Thaw meat in the microwave or in the refrigerator—never at room temperature. Cook as soon as the food has thawed. Marinating food should be refrigerated. After you remove the food from the marinade, do not use the same marinade as a sauce unless you first cook it at a rolling boil for several minutes.

COOKING TEMPERATURE

You should always cook food thoroughly to destroy the germs. The best way to be sure meat is properly cooked is to use a thermometer. While you may think color is the best barometer, neither color nor texture are reliable measures of safety. Hamburger, for example, may turn brown before it's hot enough for all bacteria to be killed; but a burger cooked to 160°F, no matter what color it is, is safe to eat.

When you cook meat, insert a meat thermometer in the thickest portion, making sure it does not touch bone. The thermometer should register 180° to 185°F for poultry and 160°F for pork. Beef (other than hamburger) is safe when cooked to a temperature of 115°F and served rare, but hamburger must always be well done. Juices should run clear when the meat is pierced. It's especially important not to partially heat food and then finish cooking it later, because half-cooked food may encourage bacterial growth.

STORING LEFTOVERS

If you've ever opened your refrigerator and discovered a bowl of furry green tufts, you know how storage problems can sneak up and surprise you. The main difficulty with leftovers is that people tend to put them away and then forget about them until weeks

REPORT FOOD POISONING

If you think someone in your family has gotten sick from eating contaminated food at a restaurant or large public gathering—especially if others have become ill also—you should report this to your city or county health department or contact www.ReportFoodPoisoning.com. Report any cases of suspected food-borne illness if you ate at a large gathering, a restaurant, or a sidewalk vendor, or if the food is a commercial product (such as canned goods, frozen food, or a supermarket-prepared salad). When making a report, include:

✗ Your name, address, and telephone number

✗ A detailed explanation of the symptoms and the suspect food

✗ When and where the food was eaten

✗ The names of people who ate the food

✗ The name and address of the place where the food was obtained

✗ For commercial food: the manufacturer's name and address and the product's lot or batch number

✗ For meat or poultry: the identity of the plant where the food was packaged (found on the USDA inspection stamp on the wrapper)

later when it's not safe to eat them anymore. We can't guarantee perfect memory, but we can recommend some ways to store food more safely. Other foods are safe from contamination from moldy foods as long as the fresh and spoiled foods are not touching.

When you're ready to put away your leftovers, divide the food into small containers to help it cool more quickly, and refrigerate it right away. Never refrigerate one large pot of hot food, because it won't be able to cool down quickly enough. Date the containers and use within three to five days. Reheat the food thoroughly; bring sauces, soups, or gravy to a boil and heat other leftovers to at least 165°F.

DEALING WITH MOLD

When there's a lot of mold growing on food, "root" threads have probably invaded throughout the food. Dangerous types of molds may contain poisonous substances in and around these threads. In some cases, toxins may have spread throughout the food.

Because mold spores from affected food can build up in your refrigerator, you should clean the inside of the appliance every few months with 1 tablespoon of baking soda dissolved in a quart of water, followed by a clear-water rinse. You should scrub off visible mold (usually black) on rubber casings using 3 teaspoons of bleach in a quart of water.

Some foods with high moisture content—like those listed below—can be contaminated below the surface, and they also may have bacteria growing along with the mold. These foods should be thrown out if they have developed mold:

× Lunch meat, bacon, hot dogs

× Cooked leftover meat and poultry

× Cooked casseroles

× Cooked grain and pasta

✖ Cottage cheese, yogurt, sour cream

✖ Soft fruits and vegetables (such as cucumbers, peaches, tomatoes)

✖ Jam: Mold on this food may produce a mycotoxin, so do not scoop out the mold and use the remaining jam.

Cheeses made with mold (such as Roquefort, blue, Brie, Camembert) should be discarded if they develop molds that are not a part of the manufacturing process, as these can be dangerous. If surface mold grows on hard cheeses such as gorgonzola and Stilton, cut off the mold at least one inch around and below the mold spot and handle like hard cheese.

If you find moldy food in your fridge, don't sniff it—this can cause breathing problems. To discard moldy food, put it into a small paper bag or wrap it in plastic and throw it away in a covered trash can that children and animals can't open. Clean the refrigerator or pantry where the food was stored, and check nearby items the moldy food might have touched. Mold spreads quickly in fruits and vegetables.

The following foods are okay to eat with mold:

✖ Hard salami and country hams: Scrub the mold off and use.

✖ Hard cheese: Cut off at least an inch around and below the mold spot, keeping the knife out of the mold itself to avoid cross-contamination; re-cover the cheese in fresh wrap.

✖ Firm fruits and vegetables: Cut off at least an inch around and below the mold spot, keeping the knife out of the mold itself. Small mold spots can be cut off fruits and vegetables with low moisture content because it's hard for mold to penetrate dense foods.

FOOD POISONING

EGG SAFETY

Throw away any cracked eggs you find in the carton; they may contain *Salmonella* bacteria. However, even an uncracked egg may contain bacteria. Since *Salmonella* is killed by heat, eggs should be cooked thoroughly. Avoid serving raw eggs (such as in Caesar salad dressing or eggnog). Eggs keep longer if you refrigerate them in the carton.

Do not store eggs on the refrigerator door. Eggs must be kept in the coldest part of the refrigerator (usually the topmost section) to prevent bacteria from multiplying.

WHEN FOOD-BORNE ILLNESS STRIKES

The time between ingestion and symptom onset varies according to the type of food poisoning, but in general symptoms usually develop:

* Within 1 to 6 hours for some types of shellfish poisoning

* Within 1 to 12 hours for most bacterial toxins

* Within 12 to 48 hours for viral and salmonella infections

Symptoms vary depending on how badly the food was contaminated but typically include nausea, vomiting, diarrhea, stomach pain, and (in severe cases) shock and collapse.

TREATMENT BASICS

Treat a mild case of food-borne illness as you would treat the flu. Provide lots of fluids (such as water, tea, bouillon, or ginger ale) to replace fluid loss from vomiting or diarrhea. Offer a soft diet, including a little salt and sugar. Most cases of food poisoning (except for botulism) aren't a serious threat to otherwise healthy children, although infants may be at higher risk. Patients usually recover within about three days.

In most cases, the greatest danger isn't from the tainted food itself, but from the body's natural response to the germs and the toxins they may produce. Vomiting and diarrhea rob the body of fluids. If the ensuing dehydration is serious enough, a child may need to be hospitalized and given intravenous fluids.

The most noted exceptions are botulism poisoning, which can lead to paralysis, and poisoning from *E. coli* bacteria, which can cause bloody stools and, in some cases, kidney failure. *E. coli* food poisoning linked to improperly cooked hamburgers killed several young children in 1993, which triggered a massive re-examination of food safety in the beef industry in the United States.

WHEN TO CALL THE DOCTOR

Food poisoning isn't a threat just to kids. You should get medical help if anyone in your family develops sudden severe vomiting, has severe or bloody diarrhea, or collapses. Suspected food poisoning should never be taken lightly if the victim is:

✖ A child

✖ Pregnant

✖ Elderly

✖ Someone with a chronic illness

✖ Someone with a compromised immune system (such as a person with AIDS or undergoing chemotherapy)

FOOD POISONING

FOOD POISONING AT A GLANCE

POISONING	MAJOR SYMPTOMS	ONSET
Anisakiasis	Abdominal pain, fever, nausea and vomiting, diarrhea	6 hours–1 week
Bacillus cereus	Diarrhea, nausea, vomiting, stomach pain	1–15 hours depending on type
Botulism	Slurred speech, double vision, muscle paralysis	6 hours–10 days
Campylobacteriosis	Headache, fever, muscle pain, diarrhea, nausea, fatigue lasting up to 10 days	1–5 days
Ciguatera	Nausea, vomiting, diarrhea, low blood pressure, severe itching, temperature reversal, numbness	6–12 hours
Cryptosporidiosis	Watery diarrhea, fever, nausea, vomiting	2–10 days
Cyclosporiasis	Watery diarrhea, cramps, gas, fever, fatigue	1 week
E. coli	Watery diarrhea, bloody diarrhea, nausea, vomiting	Hours to weeks
Giardiasis	Explosive diarrhea, foul-smelling greasy feces, stomach pain, gas, appetite loss, nausea, vomiting	1–2 weeks

POISONING	MAJOR SYMPTOMS	ONSET
Hepatitis A	Low fever, achiness, jaundice, weakness, stomach upset, pain in upper stomach	15–50 days incubation
Listeriosis	Fever, aches, headache, diarrhea, miscarriage	Days–2 months
Salmonellosis	Diarrhea, headache, fever, vomiting, cramps	6–72 hours
Shellfish poisoning	Burning mouth/extremities, nausea, vomiting, diarrhea, muscle weakness, paralysis, breathing problems	A few minutes to a few hours
Shigellosis	Fever, fatigue, diarrhea, nausea, vomiting, pain	1–2 days
Staphylococcal food poisoning	Weakness, diarrhea, cramps, vomiting	½–6 hours
Toxoplasmosis	Fever, sore throat, fatigue, rash	5–20 days
Trichinellosis	Diarrhea, nausea, vomiting, fever followed by muscle pain and stiffness	1–2 days
Vibrio	Explosive diarrhea, nausea, vomiting, cramps	4–18 hours

FOOD POISONING

ANISAKIASIS

This type of food-borne illness is caused by a parasitic worm (*Anisakis simplex*) that infests small crustaceans eaten by many kinds of fish. Humans encounter the parasite by eating improperly prepared fish (typically sushi). Anisakiasis is not a common type of food poisoning—fewer than 10 cases are diagnosed in the United States annually—but experts believe that many more cases go undiagnosed or are misdiagnosed.

The larvae of the worm are found in raw, undercooked, or insufficiently frozen fish. Pacific salmon, cod, haddock, fluke, herring, flounder, and monkfish have been known to harbor the parasite.

SYMPTOMS OF POISONING

Severe abdominal pain, fever, nausea, vomiting, and diarrhea may be experienced within six hours to one week after eating infested raw or undercooked fish. In severe cases, the pain may be misdiagnosed as appendicitis. The problem is usually diagnosed when the patient coughs up a worm.

WHAT TO DO

Any person with suspected anisakiasis should be seen by a doctor.

AT THE HOSPITAL

If the patient vomits or coughs up a worm, the disease is diagnosed by examining the worm. Otherwise, a fiber optic device may be required to examine the inside of the stomach and the first part of the small intestine. These devices include a forceps that allows the doctor to remove the worm.

Severe cases of anisakiasis are quite painful and require surgical removal of the worm, which is the only way to reduce the pain and eliminate the infestation (other than waiting for the worms to die).

BACILLUS CEREUS POISONING

This type of bacteria typically multiplies at room temperature in raw foods, producing a heat-resistant toxin most often found in refried or steamed rice. However, it also can occur in other cooked cereals, vegetables, and pasta. Experts think many episodes of this type of food-borne illness go unrecognized and unreported in the United States.

PREVENTION!

When preparing foods, especially rice, you should keep counters and other surfaces clean. Refrigerate restaurant leftovers right away and eat them immediately after reheating.

SYMPTOMS OF POISONING

These bacteria produce one of two types of symptom patterns. The problem can be dormant and symptoms—nausea, vomiting, and sometimes cramps or diarrhea—appear within one to six hours. Almost 80 percent of people with these symptoms who test positive for *B. cereus* have eaten steamed or fried rice in a Chinese restaurant. The other type takes longer to appear—between 6 and 24 hours—and causes abdominal cramps and diarrhea but very little vomiting.

WHAT TO DO

The illness is usually mild and improves without treatment.

BOTULISM

This illness, caused by ingesting the *Clostridium botulinum* bacteria, is the most potent known to mankind. Rare but quite deadly if untreated, botulism is more common in the United States than anywhere else in the world because of the popularity of home canning. Experts estimate about 20 cases of botulism occur each year in this country.

C. botulinum is a spore-forming bacterium that produces a potent neurotoxin that paralyzes muscles. Botulinum spores are found on most fresh food surfaces, but they cannot grow when exposed to oxygen. They become harmful only in an airtight environment. Spores can survive freezing, but the ideal temperature for their growth is from 78 to 98° F.

Botulism from commercial foods is rare because of strict government-enforced production standards. Most cases occur as a result of improper home canning. Still, this illness is easy to prevent by following these safety procedures provided by the National Center for Home Food Preservation:

   ✗ Consistently boil low-acid food at 212°F for 7 to 11 hours.

   ✗ Boil acid foods from 5 to 85 minutes, depending on the type of food.

   ✗ Pressure cook at 250°F for between 20 to 100 minutes, depending on the type of food.

   ✗ Boil home-canned foods for 10 minutes before eating to kill any botulism spores that may have survived the canning process.

Low-acid foods include:	Acid foods include:
All fresh vegetables	Fruits
(except for most tomatoes)	Fruit butters
Milk	Jams
Poultry	Jellies
Red meats	Marmalades
Seafood	Pickles
	Sauerkraut

Most mixtures of low-acid and acid foods are considered to be low acid, unless the recipe includes enough lemon juice, citric acid, or vinegar to make them acid.

Botulinum spores are less likely to grow in foods that are very acidic, sweet, or salty (such as canned fruit juice, jams and jellies, sauerkraut, tomatoes, or heavily salted ham). Canned foods that are much more likely to cause problems include green beans, beets, peppers, corn, and meat.

Botulism spores are tasteless, odorless, and invisible, but you can often tell that a food has been tainted because the container has lost its vacuum seal. When the spores grow, they give off gas that makes containers lose their seal, so that jars burst and cans swell. If for any reason you suspect home-canned food is spoiled, throw it away without sniffing or tasting, since botulinum toxin can be fatal even in extremely small amounts.

SYMPTOMS OF POISONING

Symptoms will start to appear anywhere from six hours to 10 days after ingestion. Symptoms including nausea, vomiting, diarrhea, stomach cramps, weakness, blurred vision, headache, difficulty in swallowing, slurred speech, drooping eyelids, dilated pupils, and paralysis. The earlier the onset of symptoms, the more severe the poisoning. Between 1976 and 1984, there were 23 deaths due to food-borne botulism in the United States. Prompt medical attention is critical because death occurs in about 70 percent of untreated cases, usually as a result of suffocation when the muscles that help with breathing become paralyzed.

Untreated illness can also paralyze arms, legs, and breathing muscles. In patients who survive, the paralysis usually improves slowly over several weeks. But untreated botulism is likely to be fatal.

DIAGNOSIS

A laboratory blood or stool test will detect *C. botulinum* toxin.

FOOD POISONING

WHAT TO DO

Suspected botulism poisoning is a medical emergency. Contact your local health department, the regional Poison Control Center (1-800-222-1222), or your health care provider if you have questions regarding a potential exposure.

AT THE HOSPITAL

If the poisoning is diagnosed early, prompt administration of antitoxin lowers the risk of death to less than 2 percent, according to the FDA. The antitoxin blocks the action of the bacteria circulating in the blood. Although antitoxin keeps the patient's condition from getting worse, it may still take many weeks for recovery, depending on the severity of the poisoning and how much time elapsed before the antitoxin was administered. The Centers for Disease Control and Prevention (CDC) in Atlanta is the only agency with the antitoxin. A patient with severe botulism may need a ventilator to survive.

INFANT BOTULISM

Infant botulism is caused by a toxin produced in an infant's intestinal tract after eating tainted food. Because this is most often caused by honey contaminated with botulinum spores, children under age one should never be fed honey.

CAMPYLOBACTERIOSIS

This food-borne illness is caused by eating raw or undercooked poultry or by drinking untreated water or unpasteurized milk.

FOOD POISONING

According to the CDC, *Campylobacter* organisms are the leading cause of bacterial diarrhea illness in the United States, affecting an estimated 2.4 million people every year—primarily children less than five years old and teens and young adults aged 15 to 29. Health care providers report more than 10,000 cases to the CDC annually. In the United States, only about 100 people (mostly the very young, the very old, and the ill) die from *Campylobacter* infection each year.

Campylobacteriosis occurs much more frequently in the summer months than in the winter. Virtually all cases occur as isolated, sporadic events, not as a part of large outbreaks. But there are exceptions. In one of the best-known outbreaks, thousands of residents in Bennington, Vermont, got sick when their town's water supply was contaminated with the bacteria.

Infection can result from handling raw poultry, eating under-cooked poultry, drinking non-chlorinated water or raw milk, or handling infected animal or human feces. Most frequently, poultry and cattle waste are the sources of the bacteria, but feces from puppies, kittens, and birds also may be contaminated. Experts estimate that up to half of all raw chicken harbors the bacteria.

SYMPTOMS OF POISONING

Infection does not lead to symptoms in every instance. If it does, symptoms typically appear between one and five days after swallowing the bacteria and include fever, headache, and muscle pain, followed by bloody diarrhea, abdominal pain, nausea, fatigue, and body aches. Symptoms usually last about two to five days, but in some cases as long as 10 days.

Long-term consequences from a *Campylobacter* infection are rare, but they include arthritis and Guillain-Barré syndrome, a disease that can cause temporary paralysis. The CDC estimates that one in every 1,000 reported campylobacteriosis cases leads to Guillain-Barré syndrome and that as many as 40 percent of Guillain-Barré syndrome cases in this country may be triggered by campylobacteriosis.

PREVENTION!

Family members should avoid drinking tainted water or unpasteurized milk. Never serve raw or undercooked chicken, poultry, or beef. Cook all poultry products thoroughly so that the meat is no longer pink, juices run clear, and the inside is cooked to 170°F for breast meat and 180°F for thigh meat. If you are served undercooked poultry in a restaurant, send it back for further cooking. When preparing foods, wash your hands with soap before and after handling raw poultry or meat, eggs, and other foods of animal origin. Prevent cross-contamination in the kitchen by using separate cutting boards for meats and other foods and carefully cleaning all cutting boards, countertops, and utensils with soap and hot water after preparing raw food of animal origin. Wash hands with soap after having contact with pet feces.

DIAGNOSIS

Many kinds of food-borne illness cause diarrhea and vomiting. Diagnosis of *Campylobacter* requires special laboratory culture procedures, which doctors may need to specifically request.

WHAT TO DO

For mild cases, rest and fluids should be all you need.

AT THE HOSPITAL

Antibiotics (such as ciprofloxacin, azithromycin, or erythromycin) must be taken at the very beginning of the illness to ease symptoms. Without treatment, stools will be infectious for several weeks, but three days of antibiotics will eliminate the bacteria. Your doctor will decide whether antibiotics are necessary.

CIGUATERA POISONING

The most commonly reported marine toxin disease in the world, ciguatera is associated with consumption of contaminated reef fish such as barracuda, grouper, and snapper. More than 300 species of tropical fish may contain ciguatoxin, an odorless, tasteless poison that cannot be destroyed by either heating or freezing. These fish are toxic at certain times of the year, when they eat a specific type of plankton that contain ciguatoxin. The Centers for Disease Control and Prevention estimates that only 2 to 10 percent of ciguatera cases in the United States are ever reported. An estimated 300 cases per 10,000 people occur each year in the U.S. Virgin Islands and the French West Indies. In Puerto Rico, 7 percent of the residents have experienced at least one episode of ciguatera in their lifetime.

PREVENTION!

If you live or vacation in areas where ciguatera outbreaks are known to occur, family members should never eat barracuda or moray eel and should be cautious with grouper and red snapper. Ask about locally caught fish associated with ciguatera. Since there is no reliable way to decontaminate ciguatoxic fish or distinguish them by smell or appearance, avoid the viscera of any reef fish.

SYMPTOMS OF POISONING

This type of food-borne illness causes both stomach and neurological symptoms, including an odd type of sensory reversal, so that cold feels hot and vice versa. Other symptoms include a tingling sensation in the lips and mouth, numbness, nausea, vomiting, stomach cramps, weakness, headache, vertigo, and—rarely—seizures or paralysis.

Symptoms may vary among individuals, different ethnic groups, and possibly with different types of fish or geographic location, but between 75 and 100 percent of people of all ages who eat the contaminated fish will experience some symptoms. In some cases, symptoms have been reported to recur after ingesting alcohol, caffeine, nuts, or any type of fish for up to three to six months following the ciguatera poisoning.

Ciguatera is rarely fatal. Any deaths that occur are usually the result of respiratory failure, circulatory collapse, or heart arrhythmias. Presently in the Pacific Ocean region, the mortality rate is less than 1 percent. Fatal cases are usually linked to ingestion of the most toxic parts of the fish (the liver, viscera, roe, and other organs).

DIAGNOSIS

There are no tests presently available for the diagnosis of ciguatera. Diagnosis is based entirely on the patient's symptoms and recent dietary history.

WHAT TO DO

Contact your doctor if you suspect someone has been sickened from eating tainted fish.

AT THE HOSPITAL

Since there is not a specific antidote for this toxin, treatment is limited to easing the symptoms.

CRYPTOSPORIDIOSIS

One of the most common causes of waterborne illness, the *Cryptosporidium parvum* parasite can be found in drinking water, as well as streams, lakes, and swimming pools, in every region of the United States. Ingestion of *Cryptosporidium* leads to cryptosporidiosis, an infection characterized by diarrhea. Once a person is infected, the parasite lives in the intestine and can be transmitted in the stool. The parasite's tough outer shell allows it to survive in the environment for long periods of time. Crypto, as it's commonly called, was not identified as a cause of human disease until 1976.

Cryptosporidium is found in soil or food, and on any surfaces contaminated with infected feces. It is commonly found in swimming pools, hot tubs, jacuzzis, fountains, lakes, rivers, springs, ponds, and streams. *Cryptosporidium* can survive for days in swimming pools, even with adequate chlorine levels, because its hard shell makes it impervious to chemicals.

SYMPTOMS OF POISONING

Some people have no symptoms at all. Others may experience watery diarrhea—the most common symptom of cryptosporidiosis—between two and 10 days after *Cryptosporidium* ingestion. Other symptoms include dehydration, weight loss, stomach cramps or pain, fever, nausea, and vomiting. Healthy individuals usually recover within one or two weeks, although symptoms may recur in cycles before the illness ends. People with a severely weakened immune system are at risk for more serious disease that could lead to life-threatening illness.

DIAGNOSIS

Testing for *Cryptosporidium* can be difficult, so the patient may need to submit several stool specimens over several days. Because these tests are not commonly performed in most laboratories, the doctor should specifically identify the test required for the parasite.

WHAT TO DO

Young children may be more susceptible to the dehydration resulting from diarrhea. They should drink plenty of fluids while ill.

Cryptosporidiosis can be very contagious. If one family member is ill, everyone needs to be extra careful about routine hygiene: Wash hands with soap and water after using the toilet or changing diapers, and before eating or preparing food. No one should swim or bathe in pools, hot tubs, streams, lakes, rivers, or the ocean for at least two weeks after diarrhea stops because *Cryptosporidium* can be passed in stool and contaminate water for several weeks. It can live for days in a treated swimming pool and be spread to other bathers.

AT THE DOCTOR'S OFFICE

The drug nitazoxanide has been approved for treatment of diarrhea caused by *Cryptosporidium* in healthy children less than 12 years old.

CYCLOSPORIASIS

Cyclospora cayetanensis is a tiny parasite that causes cyclosporiasis, an infectious illness first reported in 1979. In 1996 contaminated raspberries from Guatemala sickened people in 20 states. In 2005 Florida reported an upsurge in *Cyclospora* cases linked to local restaurants. *Cyclospora* is spread when people eat or drink food or water contaminated with infected stool, especially various types of fresh produce.

Because *Cyclospora* does not become infectious until days or weeks after being passed in a bowel movement, it probably can't be transmitted directly from one person to another. Experts don't know whether animals can pass the infection to people.

PREVENTION!

Avoiding water or food that may be contaminated with stool may help prevent *Cyclospora* infection. People who have previously been infected with this organism can become infected again.

SYMPTOMS OF POISONING

Some people who are infected with *Cyclospora* don't have any symptoms. In others, about a week after infection, *Cyclospora* causes watery diarrhea with frequent, explosive bowel movements. Other symptoms can include appetite and weight loss, bloating and gas, stomach cramps, nausea and vomiting, muscle aches, mild fever, and fatigue. If not treated, the illness may last from a few days to a month or longer.

DIAGNOSIS

Your doctor may ask you to submit several stool specimens over several days. Because *Cyclospora* tests aren't routinely done in most laboratories, your doctor should specifically request testing for the parasite.

WHAT TO DO

Patients who have diarrhea should rest and drink plenty of fluids.

AT THE DOCTOR'S OFFICE

The recommended treatment is a combination of the antibiotics trimethoprim and sulfamethoxazole (Bactrim, Septra, or Cotrim).

E. COLI POISONING

Known popularly as the "hamburger disease," this type of food-borne illness is often caused by eating undercooked hamburger tainted by the bacteria *E. coli*. Although most strains of *E. coli* are harmless and normally found in the intestines of humans and animals, a few strains can cause illness when ingested.

A particularly dangerous type is called enterohemorrhagic *E. coli* (EHEC). EHEC often causes bloody diarrhea and can lead to kidney failure in children or people with weakened immune systems. In 1982, scientists identified the first dangerous strain in the United States, *E. coli* O157:H7. (The letter-number designation refers to chemical compounds found on the bacterium's surface.) This type produces one or more related powerful toxins, which can severely damage the lining of the intestines. Other less-common types, including O26:H11 and O111:H8, also have been found in this country and can cause human disease. Cattle are the main sources of *E. coli* O157:H7, but other domestic and wild mammals also can harbor these bacteria.

E. coli bacteria and their toxins have been found in undercooked or raw hamburgers, salami, alfalfa sprouts, lettuce, scallions, well water, unpasteurized milk, apple juice, and apple cider. Swimmers have been infected by accidentally swallowing unchlorinated or underchlorinated water in swimming pools contaminated by human feces, or by swimming in sewage-contaminated bodies of water.

Fortunately, cases of this type of food-borne illness are dropping; from 1996 to 2004, the incidence of *E. coli* O157:H7 infections decreased 42 percent. The decline was linked to the federal government's recommendations that food-processing plants enhance their food safety systems. Many have applied new technologies to reduce or eliminate pathogens and have increased their testing to ensure the effectiveness of control measures. It's likely the decline also reflects livestock industry efforts to reduce *E. coli* O157:H7 in live cattle and during slaughter. Still, an estimated 10,000 to 20,000 cases occur in the United States each year, usually as a result of eating undercooked ground beef.

PREVENTION!

Hamburger is particularly prone to contamination during processing because beef from many different areas is typically mixed and ground in large amounts at once, spreading the bacteria throughout. Therefore, ground beef patties should be cooked to an internal temperature of 160°F.

Steaks and other larger cuts of meat are typically not a problem, since the bacteria remain on the outside of the meat, where it comes in direct contact with high heat during the cooking process.

Avoid unpasteurized juices, ciders, and milk. Thoroughly wash fresh fruits and vegetables—especially lettuce and scallions, and even the outside of melons— before eating.

SYMPTOMS OF POISONING

E. coli can cause severe cramps and watery diarrhea lasting for

TRAVELER'S DIARRHEA

Two types of *E. coli* found in developing countries can cause diarrhea in Americans who travel abroad. Health experts do not know how much disease some other types of *E. coli* are responsible for in the United States.

✕ Enterotoxigenic *E. coli* (ETEC) produce a toxin similar to cholera toxin. These strains typically cause "traveler's diarrhea" because they commonly contaminate food and water in developing countries.

✕ Enteropathogenic *E. coli* (EPEC) are associated with persistent diarrhea (lasting two weeks or more) and are more common in developing countries, where they can be transmitted by contaminated water or contact with infected animals.

several days, along with nausea and vomiting. Most people recover completely but complications that sometimes follow this infection can be serious.

Infection with the O157:H7 strain can lead to the development of hemolytic uremic syndrome (HUS), a life-threatening condition that destroys red blood cells and can lead to kidney failure in the very young and very old. Between 2 and 7 percent of those infected with O157:H7 end up with HUS. In the United States, HUS is the main cause of kidney failure in children.

There is no cure for HUS. About one third of those who develop it have long-term kidney trouble that can eventually require long-term dialysis. Other possible, though rare, complications are high blood pressure, blindness, and paralysis.

DIAGNOSIS

Most labs that look for *E. coli* in stool samples don't automatically test for the serious O157:H7 strain, so it's important that the doctor makes that stipulation if this organism is suspected.

WHAT TO DO

Most people with an *E. coli* infection recover within 10 days without specific treatment. There is no evidence that antibiotics help; some evidence suggests that taking them may trigger kidney problems. Anti-diarrhea medicine also should be avoided.

AT THE HOSPITAL

Hemolytic uremic syndrome is a life-threatening condition that must be treated in the hospital with blood transfusions and kidney dialysis. Even with intensive care, the death rate from HUS is between 3 and 5 percent.

GIARDIASIS

This common disease of the lower intestine is caused by contact with water, soil, or other surfaces contaminated with the protozoa *Giardia lamblia.* The parasite, which thrives in human and animal feces, is protected by an outer shell and can survive in the environment for a long time. Food can become contaminated when sewage is used as fertilizer or food handlers do not wash their hands. Since the 1990s, *Giardia* infection has become one of the most common causes of waterborne disease. Found in both drinking and recreational water, the parasites exist throughout the United States.

Giardia can be spread by accidental contact with contaminated food, beverages, or objects, such as bathroom fixtures, changing tables, or toys. It also can contaminate water in swimming pools, hot tubs, Jacuzzis, fountains, lakes, rivers, springs, ponds, or streams. Recent outbreaks in the United States have involved preschool children in day care, residents in institutions, and attendees at catered affairs and large public picnics. Many of those cases might have been prevented if food handlers had carefully washed their hands.

PREVENTION!

Giardia infection can be very contagious. If you or your children have this food-borne illness, follow these guidelines to avoid spreading the germs to others:

* Wash hands with soap and water after using the toilet, changing diapers, and before eating or preparing food.

* Don't swim in pools, hot tubs, lakes, rivers, or the ocean if you have *Giardia*, and for at least two weeks after the diarrhea ends—you can pass *Giardia* in your stool and contaminate water for several weeks after your symptoms have ended.

* Avoid fecal exposure during sexual activity.

You can try to prevent infection in the first place:

* Wash your hands thoroughly with soap and water after using the toilet and before handling or eating food.

* Wash your hands after every diaper change, especially if you work with young children and even if you wear gloves.

* Do not swim if you have diarrhea.

* Keep children in diapers out of the water.

* Avoid swallowing recreational water.

* Do not drink untreated water from shallow wells, lakes, rivers, springs, ponds, and streams; or untreated water during community-wide outbreaks of disease.

IF YOU HAVE A WELL

You should consider having your well water tested for *Giardia* if anyone using it gets sick, if your well is shallow or is at the bottom of a hill, or if the well is in a rural area where animals graze. Well water can become contaminated if animal waste seepage contaminates the ground water. This can occur if your well has cracked casings, is poorly constructed, or is too shallow.

Testing for *Giardia,* however, is expensive and difficult. Instead, you might opt for a general test of your well for fecal contamination, sampling it for the presence of coliforms or *E. coli* instead of *Giardia.* Although tests for fecal coliforms or *E. coli* won't tell you if *Giardia* is present, they will reveal whether your well water has been contaminated by fecal matter. If tests reveal fecal contamination, it's possible that the water may also be contaminated with *Giardia* or other harmful bacteria and viruses. In this case, you should stop drinking the water and contact your local water authority for instructions on how to disinfect your well.

※ Do not use untreated ice or drinking water when traveling in countries where the water supply might be unsafe.

※ Wash or peel all raw vegetables and fruits before eating.

※ Use safe, uncontaminated water to wash all food that is to be eaten raw.

※ Do not eat uncooked foods when traveling in countries with minimal water treatment and sanitation systems.

SYMPTOMS OF POISONING

Giardiasis is a mild illness and will eventually pass. In fact, about two-thirds of those infected have no symptoms. If they do occur, symptoms begin one to two weeks after infection, with explosive diarrhea, foul-smelling and greasy feces, stomach pains, gas, loss of appetite, nausea, and vomiting. In otherwise healthy people, symptoms of giardiasis may last two to six weeks. Occasionally, symptoms last longer, or the infection becomes chronic.

DIAGNOSIS

Giardiasis is diagnosed by examining a fecal sample for the presence of *Giardia*. Because this infection can be difficult to pin down, your doctor may require several stool specimens over several days. If your child attends a day care center where an outbreak is continuing despite efforts to control it, screening and treating children who have no obvious symptoms may lead to the source of the problem.

HEPATITIS A

This type of hepatitis virus is a very common cause of food-borne illness. Unlike other viruses, it can live for more than a month on kitchen countertops, kids' toys, and frozen foods and ice. In the United States, hepatitis A can occur in isolated cases or widespread epidemics. The virus causes 130,000 infections and 100 deaths each year but more than 40 percent of adults in the United States are immune as a result of a previous infection.

The disease occurs most often among school-age children and young adults, and is spread by eating food or drinking water contaminated with the virus. Inside the body, the virus multiplies and is passed in feces; it can then be carried on the hands and spread by direct contact or food handling. Hepatitis A may be found in shellfish (especially oysters), raw or undercooked food, fruits and vegetables, and well water contaminated by improperly treated sewage.

PREVENTION!

Good personal hygiene and proper sanitation can help prevent hepatitis A. Vaccines are also available for long-term prevention of infection in anyone over age two. Immune globulin is available for short-term prevention of hepatitis A virus infection in individuals of all ages.

Food handlers who know they are infected shouldn't work until they are past the infectious stage, which ends one week after first becoming jaundiced. Although federal regulations and posting of contaminated waters offer some protection, there is still a risk of the virus when eating raw shellfish.

SYMPTOMS OF POISONING

The incubation period for this virus varies from 15 to 50 days. Up to 25 percent of people who are infected won't have symptoms. Infrequently a child may have a low fever. Jaundice, which appears as a yellowing of the skin or whites of the eyes, is rare. Children over age 12 may get much sicker, with a high fever, fatigue, weakness, nausea and vomiting, stomach pain, and appetite loss. Within a few days jaundice appears.

DIAGNOSIS

Because symptoms are so similar to those of other illnesses, only a blood test can make the correct diagnosis.

WHAT TO DO

The patient should rest and eat low-fat, high-carbohydrate foods such as crackers, noodles, rice, or soup. Acetaminophen may help lower fever. Hepatitis A is much less serious than other types of hepatitis, and usually does not damage the liver as do other forms of hepatitis infection.

AT THE DOCTOR'S OFFICE

There is no drug treatment for hepatitis A. Rarely, hepatitis A can develop into a more serious form of hepatitis, completely destroying the liver cells, which can be fatal without aggressive treatment.

LISTERIOSIS

While expectant mothers are most at risk, others at high risk include the very young and the elderly, people with a weakened immune system (such as those with AIDS or patients undergoing chemotherapy), or people with diabetes, cirrhosis, asthma, or ulcerative colitis. At least 2,500 Americans become seriously ill with listeriosis each year, and 500 die. Although healthy adults and children may be infected, they don't typically get very sick.

The germ that causes listeriosis—*Listeria monocytogenes*—contaminates both soil and water, which can then contaminate vegetables grown in tainted soil or washed in unclean water. Healthy animals can carry the bacterium, leading to contaminated meats and dairy products. The bacterium also has been found in a variety of processed foods that become contaminated after processing, such as soft deli cheeses and cold cuts, and some imported deli foods. Unpasteurized milk also may contain the bacterium.

Listeria can be killed by pasteurization and cooking. However, some foods (such as hot dogs or deli meats) may be contaminated during the packaging process at the plant.

PREVENTION!

The general guidelines for the prevention of listeriosis are the same as those listed for food-borne illnesses in general. However, if you're pregnant or otherwise at high risk, you should:

× Not eat hot dogs and deli or luncheon meats.

× Not allow fluid from hot dog packages to touch other food, utensils, or kitchen surfaces.

FOOD POISONING

✖ Wash your hands before and after handling hot dogs, deli meats, and luncheon meats.

✖ Not eat soft cheeses such as feta, Brie, and Camembert; blue-veined cheeses; or Mexican-style cheeses such as queso blanco, queso fresco, and Panela unless they have labels that state they are made from pasteurized milk.

✖ Not drink unpasteurized milk or foods that contain unpasteurized milk.

✖ Refrigerate pâtés or meat spreads. It is not necessary to refrigerate canned pâtés and meat spreads.

Do not eat refrigerated smoked seafood from a deli counter or refrigerated section of a grocery store, including smoked salmon, trout, whitefish, cod, tuna, or mackerel labeled as "nova-style," "lox," "kippered," "smoked," or "jerky." Canned or shelf-stable smoked seafood are okay.

SYMPTOMS OF POISONING

Listeria causes a fever, muscle aches, and sometimes nausea or diarrhea. Infection that spreads to the nervous system may trigger headache, stiff neck, confusion, loss of balance, or convulsions. Although pregnant women exposed to listeria may experience only a mild, flu-like illness, the infection is far more serious in her unborn child, causing premature delivery, neonatal infection, miscarriage, or even stillbirth.

DIAGNOSIS

Tests of blood or spinal fluid will detect listeriosis. During pregnancy, a blood test is the most reliable way to find out if your symptoms are due to listeriosis.

Anyone in a high-risk group who develops a fever or other signs of serious illness within two months after eating a product that has been recalled because of *Listeria* contamination should inform their physician about this exposure.

AT THE DOCTOR'S OFFICE

Antibiotics given promptly to a pregnant woman can often prevent infection of the fetus or newborn. Babies with listeriosis receive the same antibiotics as adults, although a combination of antibiotics is often used until physicians are certain of the diagnosis. However, even with prompt treatment, some infections are fatal in newborns, the elderly, and those with other serious medical problems.

MAD COW DISEASE

Once confined to Great Britain, three cases of this disease in cows have now been reported in the United States. Bovine spongiform encephalopathy (BSE)—known popularly as "mad cow disease"—was first identified in British cows in 1986. It is one of a group of diseases that takes different forms in different species of animals. Cows get a type of spongiform encephalopathy called mad cow disease; humans get a spongiform encephalopathy called Creutzfeldt-Jakob disease (CJD). Humans who eat cows with mad cow disease can get a form of spongiform encephalopathy called variant-CJD (vCJD).

Mad cow disease and variant-CJD seem to be related, since they attack the brain in similar ways. These diseases are believed to be caused by prions, an unusual infectious agent that is neither bacteria nor virus. In cattle with BSE, abnormal prions initially

FOOD POISONING

occur in the small intestines and tonsils. In later stages, they are found in other tissues, including the brain and spinal cord.

The human form of mad cow disease, vCJD, is rare: As of 2006, there were 155 confirmed and probable cases of vCJD reported among the hundreds of thousands of people who may have consumed BSE-contaminated beef products around the world. The first reported case of vCJD in the United States occurred in a young woman who contracted the disease while living in the United Kingdom, and developed symptoms after moving to the United States.

The USDA surveillance program identified the first infected animal in the United States in a dairy cow in Washington in 2003; the cow was bought from a farm in Canada. A second BSE cow was identified in November 2004, and a third identified in March 2006. No cows entered the U.S. food supply. Since 1989, the USDA has banned imports of live cattle, sheep, goats, and their meat products from countries known to have BSE. Subsequently, the USDA expanded this ban to include both countries with BSE and those at risk for BSE. In 1997, the FDA prohibited (with some exceptions) the use of protein derived from the tissue of animal feed intended for cows and other hooved animals that digest their food in two steps. In 2004, the FDA issued a rule that prohibits the use of certain cattle material, because of the risk of BSE, in human food and cosmetics.

SYMPTOMS OF POISONING

First symptoms of CJD and vCJD include memory problems, with insomnia, bizarre behavior, personality changes, visual distortions, hallucinations, and dementia, ending in death.

DIAGNOSIS

Doctors use a series of tests including a specific pattern of brain waves to diagnose the condition, but the diagnosis can't be confirmed until autopsy.

SALMONELLOSIS

One of the most common types of food-borne illness, *Salmonella* poisoning is associated with a variety of foods. There are more than 2,300 strains of *Salmonella* bacteria, which multiply quickly at room temperature. *Salmonella enteritidis* and *S. typhimurium* are the two types of these bacteria most commonly found in the United States.

Most, but not all *salmonella* strains are relatively harmless. A strain of *S. typhimurium* called Definitive Type 104 (DT104) that is resistant to several antibiotics normally used to treat *Salmonella* has been identified in the United States.

Salmonellosis has occurred in small, contained outbreaks in the general population and in large outbreaks in hospitals, restaurants, and institutions that care for sick children and the elderly. Every year, the CDC receives reports of at least 40,000 cases of salmonellosis in the United States, but estimates that unreported cases put the number to at least 1.4 million people. About 1,000 people die of salmonella poisoning each year.

Salmonella bacteria occur in raw poultry, eggs, and beef, and sometimes on unwashed fruit. Food prepared on surfaces that previously touched raw meat or meat products can become contaminated with the bacteria. There also have been reports of several cases of salmonellosis that occurred from eating raw alfalfa sprouts grown in contaminated soil. *Salmonella* infection also may occur after handling reptiles such as snakes, turtles, and lizards.

People can be infected with a chronic *Salmonella* infection but show no symptoms, and they can spread the disease by handling food with unwashed hands. Health care experts recommend that people who know they have salmonellosis should not prepare food or pour beverages for others until laboratory tests show they no longer carry the bacteria.

FOOD POISONING

PREVENTION!

Salmonellosis can be prevented by following the general prevention guidelines beginning on page 198.

SYMPTOMS OF POISONING

Symptoms are most severe in infants, the elderly, and people with chronic disease. People with AIDS are particularly vulnerable to salmonellosis and often suffer from recurring episodes. Within six hours to three days after infection, symptoms usually begin with diarrhea, fever, stomach cramps, and headache. These symptoms, along with nausea, loss of appetite, and vomiting, usually last for up to a week. Diarrhea can be severe and require hospitalization. Unless treated properly, *Salmonella* bacteria can escape from the intestine and spread by blood to other organs, sometimes leading to death.

DIAGNOSIS

Laboratory stool testing can identify *Salmonella*.

WHAT TO DO

In most cases the infection clears up on its own without treatment. It is important, however, to drink plenty of fluids if there is nausea or vomiting.

AT THE DOCTOR'S OFFICE

If a patient has severe diarrhea, intravenous fluids may be needed. If the infection spreads from the intestines into the bloodstream, it can be treated with antibiotics such as ampicillin.

SHELLFISH POISONING

Shellfish poisoning is caused by a group of toxins produced by the underwater plankton on which the shellfish feed. The toxins are accumulated and sometimes metabolized by the shellfish.

There are four different types of poisoning that can be caused by eating contaminated shellfish: amnesic (ASP), associated with eating mussels; diarrheic (DSP), associated with eating mussels, oysters, and scallops; neurotoxic (NSP), associated with eating shellfish harvested along the Florida coast and the Gulf of Mexico; and paralytic (PSP), usually associated with eating mussels, clams, cockles, and scallops.

Amnesic shellfish poisoning (ASP). This type of shellfish poisoning was first identified by public health authorities in 1987, when 156 cases were diagnosed as a result of eating cultured blue mussels harvested off Prince Edward Island; 22 individuals were hospitalized and three elderly patients eventually died.

Diarrheic shellfish poisoning (DSP). The occurrence of DSP in Europe is sporadic, continuous, and presumably widespread, but DSP poisoning has not been confirmed in U.S. seafood. However, the organisms that produce DSP are found in U.S. waters. An outbreak of DSP was recently confirmed in eastern Canada.

Neurotoxic shellfish poisoning (NSP). Outbreaks of NSP are sporadic and continuous along the Gulf coast of Florida and have been reported in North Carolina and Texas.

Paralytic shellfish poisoning (PSP). This is caused by eating tainted mussels, clams, and scallops, or broth from cooked shellfish. PSP is associated with relatively few outbreaks, probably because of the thorough control programs in the United States that prevent human exposure to toxic shellfish, but PSP outbreaks did occur in Massachusetts and Alaska in June 1990. PSP can be a serious public health problem; for example, a Guatemala outbreak of 187 cases in 1987 killed 26 people who ate tainted clam soup. The outbreak led to the establishment of a control program over shellfish harvested in Guatemala.

PREVENTION

To prevent poisoning outbreaks, state health departments during certain times of the year routinely test samples of shellfish. If contamination is found, affected areas are quarantined and sale

FOOD POISONING

of the shellfish is prohibited. There's no way to tell just by looking at the water whether toxic plankton are present. PSP toxin cannot be killed by freezing.

SYMPTOMS OF POISONING

Eating contaminated shellfish results in a wide variety of symptoms, depending upon the toxins, their concentrations in the shellfish, and the amount of contaminated shellfish eaten. Cases are often misdiagnosed and are often not reported.

ASP: Life-threatening symptoms include gastrointestinal symptoms within 24 hours and neurological symptoms within 48 hours, with dizziness, headache, seizures, disorientation, short-term memory loss, respiratory difficulty, and coma. Symptoms are particularly serious in the elderly, and can mimic Alzheimer's disease. All fatalities to date have involved elderly patients. Long-term memory loss can occur as a result of permanent brain damage.

DSP: Symptoms begin within 30 minutes to two or three hours after eating, depending on how much shellfish was consumed, and include severe diarrhea, nausea, vomiting, abdominal cramps, and chills.

NSP: The toxin attacks the nervous system and triggers both stomach and neurological problems within a few minutes to hours after ingestion. It causes tingling or numb lips, tongue, and throat; muscular aches; dizziness; hot/cold sensory reversal; diarrhea; and vomiting. Recovery is complete with very few aftereffects, and no fatalities have been reported.

PSP: The toxin attacks the nervous system and triggers both stomach and neurological problems within a few minutes to hours after ingestion. Symptoms may include nausea, vomiting, diarrhea, abdominal pain, muscular aches, a sensation of floating, dizziness, headache, difficulty speaking or swallowing, and paralysis. With good medical care, recovery is complete with very few long-term effects.

FOOD POISONING

There is no known antidote for any type of shellfish poisoning, and no drug has proven effective against the more serious forms. Treatment is limited to treating the symptoms.

SHIGELLOSIS

Shigellosis (also known as bacillary dysentery) is an infectious disease caused by four main types of *Shigella* bacteria: *Shigella dysenteriae, S. flexneri, S. boydii,* and *S. sonnei.* The most common type in the United States is *S. sonnei.* The U.S. Centers for Disease Control and Prevention estimates that more than 400,000 cases of shigellosis occur every year nationwide.

A person can be infected by:

× Eating food contaminated by infected handlers who don't properly wash their hands after using the bathroom.

× Eating vegetables grown in fields containing sewage.

× Eating food contaminated by flies bred in infected feces

× Swimming in or swallowing contaminated water.

Even if you have no symptoms of shigellosis, you can still pass the bacteria to others, because an extremely small number of bacteria (just 10 to 100) can transmit the infection. If you know you have shigellosis, you shouldn't prepare food or pour beverages for others until laboratory tests show you no longer carry the bacteria.

SYMPTOMS OF POISONING
Usually beginning within a day or two after exposure, symptoms

include fever, fatigue, watery or bloody diarrhea, nausea, vomiting, and stomach pain.

WHAT TO DO

Symptoms are usually mild enough that simple rest and fluids are all that's recommended. All symptoms usually pass within a week. Antidiarrheal medicines may make the illness worse. People usually recover from diarrhea on their own, although their bowel habits may not return to normal until several months later.

AT THE DOCTOR'S OFFICE

For severe symptoms, your family doctor may prescribe an antibiotic such as ampicillin or ciprofloxacin. *S. dysenteriae* type 1 produces *Shigilla* toxin, which can lead to life-threatening hemolytic uremic syndrome (HUS), a serious condition that can cause kidney failure.

STAPHYLOCOCCAL POISONING

This type of food poisoning is caused by a toxin produced by *Staphylococcus* bacteria (usually *S. aureus*) found on the skin and in the nose, mouth, and throat of many healthy people. Food can become tainted when someone with the bacteria handles food with bare hands, especially after touching the face or mouth. If the contaminated food isn't then cooked thoroughly or properly kept hot or cold, the bacteria can produce a toxin that will sicken anyone who eats it. Foods commonly tainted in this way include ham, poultry, filled pastries, custard, egg salad, and potato salad.

PREVENTION

Touch food with bare hands as little as possible, and never handle food with your bare hands after touching your face. If you do touch your face while preparing food, wash your hands again. If you have an exposed infection (such as a cut on the hand), you should not prepare or handle food at all.

SYMPTOMS OF POISONING

Weakness, cramps, diarrhea, vomiting, and nausea are experienced beginning 30 minutes to six hours after eating the contaminated food. Symptoms typically fade away without treatment within a day.

DIAGNOSIS

The quick onset of the symptoms usually confirms the infection, but your family doctor may order tests to rule out other conditions.

WHAT TO DO

Drink lots of fluids to help the body replace those lost due to diarrhea and vomiting. There is no medicine to cure staphylococcal food poisoning.

TOXOPLASMOSIS

Toxoplasmosis is caused by the parasite *Toxoplasma gondii,* which can be transmitted by eating undercooked meat, drinking contaminated water, or touching infected cat feces. It is most serious in pregnant women, because it can lead to birth defects. The highest risk occurs if the mother is infected during the first six months of pregnancy. Severe symptoms also can occur in anyone whose immune system is severely weakened by HIV/AIDS, chemotherapy, or a recent organ transplant.

PREVENTION!

If you're planning to get pregnant, your doctor may test you for *Toxoplasma*. If the test is positive, you've already been infected at some point in your life and you probably don't need to worry about passing the infection to your baby. If the test is negative, you should take necessary precautions to avoid infection. This would include not cleaning your cat's litter box and wearing gloves if you garden. If you're already pregnant, you and your doctor should discuss your risk for toxoplasmosis.

SYMPTOMS OF POISONING

Most people who become infected with *Toxoplasma* don't know it. Between five and 20 days after exposure, slight lymph node swelling may appear, along with a low fever, sore throat, fatigue, or slight body rash. Infants are much more severely affected than their infected mothers and can be born with eye problems, jaundice, water on the brain, or mental retardation.

DIAGNOSIS

Toxoplasmosis is diagnosed by a blood test.

WHAT TO DO

Treatment usually is not needed in an otherwise healthy person who isn't pregnant.

AT THE DOCTOR'S OFFICE

Medications are available for pregnant women or anyone with a weakened immune system.

TRICHINELLOSIS

Associated with eating raw or undercooked pork or wild game meats such as bear, cougar, fox, wolf, seal, or walrus, this type of potentially fatal food poisoning was once quite common but is now fairly rare. There are about 40 cases a year, according to the National Institutes of Health. Infection occurs when people ingest meat contaminated with the larvae of a parasitic worm, *Trichinella*. The number of cases has dropped because of laws against feeding raw meat to hogs, more emphasis on freezing pork (which kills the worms), and increased public awareness of the danger of eating undercooked pork products.

PREVENTION!

Cook pork products until the juices run clear, or until an internal temperature of 170° F is reached. Cook wild game meat thoroughly; freezing wild game meats even for a long period may not kill all the worms. If you do your own meat grinding, you should clean the grinder thoroughly. Curing, drying, smoking, or microwaving meat does not always kill the worms.

SYMPTOMS OF POISONING

Mild cases of trichinellosis may not cause any symptoms; the severity of problems that do occur depends on how many infectious worms were in the meat that was consumed. Stomach pain, diarrhea, nausea, vomiting, along with fatigue and fever, begin one or two days after infestation. Within two weeks to two months after eating contaminated meat, these initial symptoms may be followed by chills and aching joints, constipation or diarrhea, cough, headaches, eye swelling, fever, itchy skin, and muscle pain.

A severe infection may cause difficulty with coordination, and may eventually affect breathing or the heart. Very severe cases can be fatal. Most people with a mild case get better within a month or two, although they may still struggle with diarrhea or feeling tired and weak for some time.

WHAT YOU CAN DO

Treat symptoms; call a doctor if symptoms are severe.

AT THE DOCTOR'S OFFICE

Your doctor will prescribe one of several safe and effective prescription drugs as quickly as possible. A doctor typically decides to treat this condition based on the patient's symptoms, a history of exposure to raw or undercooked meat, and positive lab tests.

FOOD POISONING

VIBRIO

This type of food-borne illness is caused by eating fish or shellfish contaminated with *Vibrio parahaemolyticus* bacteria. A cousin of the bacteria that cause cholera, these naturally occurring organisms live in brackish salt water along coasts; they are commonly found in waters where oysters are cultivated. When just the right salinity and temperature conditions occur, *V. parahaemolyticus* thrives.

Occasional outbreaks of *Vibrio* poisoning occur in the United States when people eat undercooked or raw contaminated oysters. Less frequently, this organism also can cause a skin infection if an open wound is exposed to warm seawater.

Once inside the body, the bacteria attach themselves to the small intestine, where they secrete an as-yet-unidentified toxin. Anyone who eats raw or improperly cooked contaminated fish or shellfish is at risk for *Vibrio* (especially during warmer months). Improper refrigeration of the contaminated seafood allows the bacteria to grow, increasing the risk of infection.

Not all states require that *V. parahemolyticus* infections be reported to the state health department, but in the states that do (including Alabama, Florida, Louisiana, and Texas) about 30 to 40 cases of *V. parahaemolyticus* infections are reported each year.

PREVENTION!

Most infections caused by *V. parahaemolyticus* in the United States could be prevented by thoroughly cooking oysters, and by not exposing open wounds to warm seawater. When an outbreak is traced to a particular oyster bed, health officials typically close the area to harvesting until conditions no longer favor the growth of this organism.

SYMPTOMS OF POISONING

Chills, cramps and diarrhea, nausea and vomiting, headache, and fever may begin to appear four to 18 hours after ingestion.

DIAGNOSIS

Vibrio organisms can be isolated from cultures of stool, wounds, or blood.

WHAT YOU CAN DO

Drink plenty of liquids to replace fluids lost through diarrhea. Otherwise, treatment is not necessary in most cases.

AT THE DOCTOR'S OFFICE

There is no evidence that antibiotic treatment is effective, although in cases of severe or prolonged illness, antibiotics such as tetracycline, ampicillin, or ciprofloxicin may be prescribed.

FOOD POISONING

9

KEEP BABY SAFE

POISONS IN THE NURSERY AND PLAYROOM

Setting up a nursery is an exciting time. You'll spend lots of time comparing paint and wallpaper swatches, choosing a crib and changing table, and finding just the right toys and decorations for your soon-to-be little one. You want everything to be perfect! But it will never be perfect until you also make sure your baby's room is as safe as possible.

Babies and toddlers are not tiny adults, and it's important to understand this difference—especially when dealing with toxic substances in the nursery or playroom. Because of your child's low body weight, it takes a very small amount of a toxic material to cause harm. And because infants and toddlers grow so quickly, chemicals to which they are exposed can be absorbed into their body tissues more quickly and in higher concentrations than in adults. In particular, a baby's brain is extremely vulnerable to poisons in the environment, since the brain continues to grow and develop for the first few years. At the same time, the organs responsible for detoxifying harmful substances—the intestines, liver, and kidneys—aren't fully developed in early childhood.

Surprising as it may be, most new decorating items such as carpets, wallpaper, and even furniture contain chemicals that can be harmful to your baby's development. Particularly troublesome is lead contamination. Lead can be found almost anywhere in the home, especially in older houses.

NONTOXIC SUBSTANCES IN BABY'S NURSERY AND PLAYROOM

There are some items commonly found in the nursery or playroom that you can be assured are perfectly harmless when chewed or swallowed by babies and young children. Among the most common are:

Baby oil	Kaolin (in clay)
Blackboard chalk	Lanolin (in ointments, etc.)
Bubble bath	Modeling clay
Castor oil	Petroleum jelly
Diaper rash ointment	Soap
Graphite (in "lead" pencils)	Teething rings
Hand creams, lotions	Watercolor paint

KEEPING BABY'S ROOM CLEAN

Of course you want your baby's bedroom to be spic and span, but infants can be very sensitive to the ammonia, chemicals, and fragrances in commercial cleaners. There are many nontoxic cleaners to choose from that are both safe and effective.

SOME MOMS SWEAR BY....

* ½ cup of white vinegar mixed into 1 gallon of water to clean surfaces, glass, and windows

* Paste of white vinegar and salt for a good surface cleaner

* 4 tablespoons of baking soda mixed into 1 quart of warm water for a general cleaner

Remember to keep windows wide open while you're cleaning to let lots of fresh air into the room, even in winter. An air purifier can help minimize irritants and air pollutants.

ART SUPPLIES

When buying art supplies, look for products that are safe for children; many art supplies used for hobbies and crafts contain lead, mercury, or other toxic chemicals. Buy only products that are labeled "conforms to ASTM D4236" and that bear the seal of the Arts and Creative Materials Institute (ACMI). If a company doesn't use the rating system, it's best to consider the material potentially toxic, or contact the company for more information. You should buy only products with the ACMI Non-Toxic Seals CP, AP, and HL [Non-Toxic] for children under age six, the physically or mentally

NURSERY

handicapped, and anyone who can't read or understand the safety labeling on product packages.

Products that have been found to be safe after a toxicological evaluation by a medical expert bear the ACMI certification seal. They are certified to contain no materials in sufficient quantities to be toxic or injurious to humans, including children.

Smell is not a good indicator of how toxic an art material may be. Sometimes a product (such as markers) can have a strong odor and yet still be nontoxic. On the other hand, something that has no smell or that smells sweet could be very poisonous. Many dusty or dry products, such as chalk, powdered tempera, and many pastels, are nontoxic even if inhaled. On the other hand, some dust-causing products, such as many dry clays, can be poisonous.

SAFE ART SUPPLIES

Many of the best-known art supply companies that market to children are ACMI-approved, including Binney & Smith (Crayola), Rose Art, Sanford (Sharpie), and Prang. For a complete list of all ACMI-approved products, visit this web site: www.acminet.org/CPListSearch.html

WHAT TO DO

If you suspect your child has eaten an art product, first read the label and follow any instructions that may appear there. If the product bears a warning, call the Poison Control Center (1-800-222-1222) and have the package in front of you so you can describe the ingredients and relate any first aid directions printed on the label. If the product has a nontoxic seal from the Art and Creative Materials Institute (ACMI), you can consider it safe.

PREVENTION!

Never allow your kids to use any product for painting on their skin

NURSERY

or in cooking unless it's clear that the material was meant to be used this way. When cleaning up or organizing your child's bedroom or playroom, don't transfer art materials to other containers—you'll lose the valuable safety information that's on the product package.

To prevent skin contact or inhalation of fumes, keep your baby well away from art materials such as paints, pastels, and enamels, as well as solder and cleaning supplies such as turpentine. Constant low-level exposure of children to these substances can potentially lead to other detrimental health effects.

LEAD POISONING

Lead paint found in older homes is one of the leading sources of lead poisoning for children in North America. Although lead paint was commonly used in American homes until 1978, the highest concentration of lead in paint is found in homes built before 1950. Unfortunately, lead paint remnants in old homes and buildings today still pose a significant threat to America's children. High lead levels in the body can accumulate from repeated exposure, and can cause irreversible mental and behavior problems in children.

Fortunately, U.S. lead poisoning cases have decreased by about 86 percent since the late 1970s as a result of widespread publicity alerting parents to the dangers of lead-based paints. However, research reveals that African-American, immigrant, and poor children continue to have higher levels of lead in their blood than other kids.

Children by their mere size are more sensitive than adults to the side effects of lead, and children under age five are particularly vulnerable for a variety of reasons. First, they tend to put everything into their mouths, which puts them at higher risk. Second, once they are exposed to lead, their still-developing

NURSERY

young bodies and brains are more vulnerable to damage. In fact, lead poisoning has been linked to lower IQ scores in children exposed to even low levels of lead.

The most common cause of lead poisoning is from interior wall paint in older homes. Residual lead in old paint remains active and can contaminate dust, soil, water, and air in the vicinity of older homes. Children have been known to get contaminated by putting hands or toys tainted with lead dust in their mouths, eating lead paint chips that peel off walls, and chewing on window sills and door frames.

Children also have been poisoned by lead from numerous other sources:

Parent's Work Environment

Adults may track lead dust home from the workplace on their clothes, hands, hair, and shoes. Jobs that carry risk of exposure to lead include house painting or wallpapering older homes, home renovation, furniture refinishing, lead smelting or mining, firearms instruction, car repair, battery manufacturing or recycling, and construction work on bridges, tunnels, or elevated highways.

Parent's Hobby

Certain hobbies may contaminate the home with lead dust or fumes, or contaminate a parent's clothes, hands, hair, or shoes. Examples include target shooting, making ceramics, and melting lead for homemade musket balls or fishing tackle. Stained glass artists may use lead solder, as well as solid lead to wrap around individual pieces of glass and to frame artwork.

Contaminated Soil

Although lead was completely phased out of gasoline by 1995, lead particles emitted in engine exhaust still persist in soil near some major roadways. Also, deteriorating exterior lead paint may contaminate the soil around old homes. Children who play in bare soil risk exposure to lead, and family members may track contaminated soil into the home on their shoes.

NURSERY

Ceramics

Lead is used in some ceramic glazes, and improperly fired glazes and deteriorating glazes on ceramic mugs, bowls, and dishes may leach lead into food and beverages, especially after prolonged contact or if the food is hot or acidic. In the United States, most glazes for ceramic products contain lead but are safe because they have been properly formulated and fired to prevent the release of toxic amounts of metal into foods. The FDA, however, does not regulate handmade items. Ceramics bought in foreign countries and items not intended for food use also may leach high levels of lead.

Lead Solder

Solders with varying concentrations of lead are used in the electronics industry and in making stained glass. Some people use lead solder illegally to make homemade fishing tackle or in home plumbing projects. Weights and sinkers are small, smooth, and easily swallowed by curious children, especially when imitating adults who use their teeth to manipulate the tackle. Those made out of lead can cause problems for humans, birds, fish, and other animals if swallowed. Many states have enacted restrictions and bans of lead fishing sinkers, because the lead poses an environmental threat. People who make their own wine or liquor may use stills soldered with lead, which can result in lead leaching into the beverage. In 1995 the FDA banned lead-soldered food cans, but some may still occasionally be imported illegally into the United States and sold, especially in ethnic grocery stores. Soldering is messy and creates tiny fragments and dust-sized particles of lead, as well as lead fumes.

Drinking Water

Most public water sources are routinely tested and don't exceed the Environmental Protection Agency (EPA) lead limits of less than 15 parts per billion (ppb). For bottled water, the level is 5 ppb. However, water may become contaminated if it flows through old lead-soldered pipes or lead-containing faucets inside old buildings. Lead levels are highest in water left standing in pipes for more than a few hours, and in hot or acidic water. This is why you should use cold water from taps for cooking, especially in older homes with lead-soldered pipes. You should replace lead-soldered pipes and lead-containing faucets.

PAINT SENSE

If you're going to paint baby's room, be sure to have the decorating completed several weeks before your due date so all of the odors and fumes will have had a chance to dissipate. Also keep in mind that you should not be painting when you're pregnant; the fumes could affect your baby. Delegate that chore to your spouse or a friend.

Costume/Toy Jewelry

Cheap jewelry marketed to children (often sold in vending machines) has been the source of several documented cases of acute lead poisoning. Children readily chew or suck on the items, or unintentionally swallow them. Although toy jewelry containing lead is a banned hazardous substance, such items may illegally be on the market. Imported jewelry is especially suspect. If you're not certain where these items come from, don't let your children wear or play with them.

Curtain Weights

Sewn into the hem of curtains or drapes, some curtain weights are made of lead and are small enough to be swallowed even by a child. If you notice tears in your curtains, remove them and throw them out.

Artist Oil Paint

One color of fine art oil paint, "flake white," contains lead carbonate. Many artists feel there is no substitute for this product, which enhances a painting's durability. As a result, artists lobbied successfully for its exemption from the U.S. Consumer Product Safety Commission's 1977 ban on lead paint. Artists with small children should be careful to keep this product out of curious hands.

Vinyl Mini-Blinds

Vinyl mini-blinds made before 1997 may contain lead. Over time, exposure to heat and sunlight deteriorates the vinyl and lead dust forms on the surface. Blinds made with lead were recalled and banned by the Consumer Product Safety Commission in 1997, but prior to that date millions of them were sold and may still be in many U.S. homes. If you have vinyl mini-blinds that were installed before 1997, have them replaced. At the very least, make sure they're not installed in the nursery!

Pool Cue Chalk

The use of lead as a coloring agent in pool cue chalk is often denied by the industry. Nevertheless, one study in 1996 did conclude that three of 23 brands of pool cue chalk tested contained lead; one had as much as 7,000 parts per million (ppm).

Antique Toys

The Consumer Product Safety Commission continually screens newly produced toys for hazardous substances including lead or lead paint. Vintage toys may contain lead—especially toy cars, planes, and trucks; painted toys; and toy soldiers or other figurines.

Tin-Coated Lead Foil on Wine Bottles

Wine bottled prior to 1996 may have lead foil covering the cork. Studies show that some contamination of the wine can occur when it is poured. Children may ingest lead if they chew or swallow the foil. In 1996, the FDA banned the use of lead foil on wine bottles sold in the United States.

NURSERY

Leaded Crystal

Like ceramics, leaded crystal can leach lead into food or beverages, especially following prolonged contact or if the beverage is acidic. Experts advise against storing beverages in a lead crystal container or routinely drinking from crystal. As a result of research showing that lead can leach into wine from lead crystal, leading wine-glass manufacturers such as Wedgwood, Waterford, and Rosenthal reworked some of their lead crystal wine glass lines to lower their lead oxide contents. However, never feed your baby with a bottle made out of lead crystal.

Kohl

Kohl is an ancient black cosmetic still used by some women in the Middle East, Asia, and Africa. It often contains ground *galena,* a mineral that is a source of lead. Some cultures also put kohl on the umbilical stump of newborns, or use it to decorate the eyes and faces of children. Kohl is illegal in the United States, yet it may be found in some ethnic shops or available for purchase online. Travelers sometimes bring kohl home to the United States, unaware of its dangers.

Mexican Candies

Studies have found high levels of lead in many Mexican candies, especially those containing tamarind or chili powder. Ink used to print the wrappers has also been shown to contain dangerous amounts of lead. For a comprehensive and informative report on lead in Mexican candy, including links to test results and a full color index of types of candies that tested positive for lead, visit the Web site of the Southern California newspaper, *The Orange County Register*: www.ocregister.com/investigations/2004/lead/part1.shtml

Projectiles (Bullets)

Lead has been used to make projectiles since the mid-fifteenth century. Its widespread availability, malleability, and high density continue to make it ideal for this purpose. Today most bullets for shotguns, handguns, and rifles are made of a lead core surrounded by a copper or steel jacket to protect the lead from changing shape at high speeds. Economical solid lead bullets are also available, as are traditional lead musket balls. Curious young children will readily swallow projectiles. Buckshot (small balls of lead used by hunters) may remain in cooked game and be unintentionally eaten.

SYMPTOMS OF POISONING

Lead can harm virtually every system in the human body. It is particularly harmful to the developing brain and nervous system of fetuses and young children. In many cases, however, there are no visible symptoms of elevated blood lead levels or lead poisoning.

If symptoms do occur, they may include fatigue, stomach pains, headaches, changes in personality or a drop in grades, and pain in hands, feet, muscles, or joints.

DIAGNOSIS

The only way to be sure whether your child has been exposed to lead is with a quick and easy blood test. Every child who meets specific criteria set by the Centers for Disease Control and Prevention should be tested. If you don't have a doctor to advise you, the U.S. Department of Health and Human Services can help: call 212-BAN-LEAD to find out how to get your child tested at your local health department. Many private insurance policies cover the cost of testing for blood lead levels; children covered by Medicaid are eligible for free screening. The cost of a blood lead test generally ranges from $10 to $75, plus the charge for an office visit. If your child is at risk for lead poisoning and you are unable to pay for testing, contact your local health department for assistance.

WHAT TO DO

The best treatment for lead poisoning is to stop the exposure. Removing the lead from your child's environment will help ensure a decline in blood lead levels.

NURSERY

AT THE DOCTOR'S OFFICE

Appropriate treatment depends on the child's blood lead level. If the level is only a bit high, your doctor may simply advise measures to reduce lead exposure and arrange to have the level retested later. In other cases, immediate medical treatment may be required. Medical treatment primarily consists of chelating agents (medications that bind to lead and help remove it from the body), which can be administered by mouth or intravenously. The longer your child was exposed to lead, the greater the chance that there could be health consequences. In some cases, medications are used to lower blood-lead levels.

PREVENTION!

You'll want to keep your children away from peeling paint, especially if your home was built before 1978. Wash your children's hands before they eat, after they play outdoors, and before they go to sleep—and wash your own hands before preparing food. Make sure that their diet is nutritious and that they receive the iron, calcium, and vitamins needed for growth and development.

To temporarily reduce lead paint and dust in older homes, clean the floors, windowsills, and window wells at least twice a week with a trisodium phosphate detergent available at hardware stores. Sponges used for this purpose shouldn't be used for anything else. Move cribs and playpens away from chipped or peeling paint, mantels, windowsills, and doors. Replace or strip furniture that may contain finish with lead paint.

When cooking, run the cold water tap for at least a minute before drawing water for use. Never use hot water from the faucet to make baby formula or for cooking; that water can more readily absorb lead from pipes. Never boil water thinking that you'll eliminate lead this way; in fact, boiling only concentrates the lead.

Be wary of imported canned food; the seams of the cans may be soldered with lead, which can seep into the contents. In addition, don't store acidic food (such as orange juice or tomatoes) in ceramic or crystal containers, which may contain lead glaze.

It's also important to protect your children outdoors, where lead can contaminate the soil, water, and outdoor structures painted before 1978. Don't let children play under bridges or near highways and heavily traveled roads. If your property soil tests high in lead, cover it with clean soil and seed or sod.

WHO SHOULD BE SCREENED?

Screening for elevated blood lead levels is recommended for children up to age two if they meet any of the criteria listed here. In addition, children aged three to five who haven't been previously tested and meet any of the criteria also should be tested

× Eligible for, or receiving, Medicaid or Women, Infants, and Children (WIC) benefits

× Living in a ZIP code that's considered to be high risk, based on age of housing and other factors. Check with your local health department about high-risk areas

× Living in or regularly visiting a house built before 1950

× Living in or regularly visiting a house or day care center built between 1950 and 1978 that is undergoing renovations or where paint is peeling or chipping

× Living with or regularly visiting a sibling, housemate, or playmate with lead poisoning

× Living with an adult whose job or hobby involves exposure to lead

× Living near an active lead smelter, battery recycling plant, or other industry likely to release lead

NURSERY

FOR MORE INFORMATION ON LEAD

U.S. Department of Environmental Protection
(718) 699-9811
For information about testing your water for lead

The EPA's National Lead Information Center
(800) 424-5323

U.S. Environmental Protection Agency
www.epa.gov/lead/index.html

Centers for Disease Control and Prevention
(404) 639-3534
www.cdc.gov/lead

TALCUM POWDER

Talcum powder, which contains the mineral talc, is potentially harmful to infants, and it should never be used as a powder during diaper changing. Inhaled talcum powder causes serious breathing complications. Talcum powder is toxic if swallowed. How well a baby recovers after exposure to talcum powder depends on how quickly the baby is treated and how much powder was inhaled or swallowed.

SYMPTOMS OF POISONING
Inhaling talcum powder can cause twitching, fever, cough and breathing problems, convulsions, and collapse.

WHAT TO DO

Call the regional Poison Control Center (1-800-222-1222) immediately if your baby may have inhaled or swallowed talcum powder. If the powder gets on the baby's skin, wash it off immediately.

AT THE HOSPITAL

If your baby has inhaled the powder and is showing any of the
symptoms of poisoning, the doctor may administer oxygen and
take a chest x-ray. In the worst cases, the doctor may need to
insert a breathing tube, or put your baby in the intensive care
unit in a tent filled with mist.

KEEPING BABY CLEAN

All you really need to keep your baby clean is a little
warm water and a washcloth. If you want to use soap,
select only mild soaps and fragrance-free shampoos
specifically made for baby. Use only products labeled
"hypoallergenic" and ointments with simple ingredients. If you choose products developed specifically for
infants and made by reputable companies, you and your
baby will be fine.

NURSERY

10

PROTECT YOUR PETS

SAFEGUARDS FOR THE CURIOUS

Your kids aren't the only family members especially vulnerable to poisoning—pets are also at increased risk. In particular, dogs are notorious for getting accidentally poisoned, since they are curious and like to eat almost anything. The three most common causes of serious poisonings in dogs are snail bait, rat poison, and antifreeze. Any of these can be life threatening. Remember, treating a pet for poisoning is often prolonged and expensive—and a good outcome isn't guaranteed. It's much better to prevent the poisoning in the first place.

If you suspect that your pet has been poisoned, the fastest and best way to react is to *immediately* call the Pet Poison Control Center's HELPLINE or the American Society for the Prevention of Cruelty to Animals' (ASPCA) national Animal Poison Control Center. While a veterinarian should be able to help, not all vets are toxicological experts. If you suspect a pet poisoning, don't delay: Call immediately! Prompt attention may make a crucial difference to your pet. Even if you think you know what to do to help your pet, you should get expert advice before attempting to treat an animal yourself.

> Have the phone numbers of these poison control centers, your regular veterinarian, and your local emergency veterinary service posted in a prominent place near the phone.
>
> ASPCA Animal Poison Control Center   888-426-4435
>
> Pet Poison HELPLINE   800-213-6680

For more than 25 years, the ASPCA Animal Poison Control Center—an allied agency of the University of Illinois—has been giving advice about pet poisons. Staffed by 25 veterinarians, the center includes six board-certified veterinary toxicologists and 10 certified vet technicians. The center is available 24 hours a day, seven days a week to give help to callers—both pet owners and veterinarians. Staffers responded to more than 95,000 cases in 2004. Armed with information on more than 850,000 cases involving pesticides, drugs, plants, metals, and other exposures, they can make specific diagnostic and treatment recommendations.

A call costs $50 per case, which will be charged to a major credit card. When you call, be ready to give your name, address, and phone number; information about the suspected poison, including how long since your pet got into the material; symptoms; and details about your pet (species, breed, age, sex, and weight). At your request, staffers will also consult with your vet and make as many follow-up calls as necessary.

The Pet Poison HELPLINE is a nationwide 24-hour service available to pet owners and veterinary professionals who need help treating a potentially poisoned pet. Run by the Pet Poison Control Center, it's staffed with veterinary health professionals and clinical toxicologists who each have more than 28 years of experience and expertise. The help line offers treatment advice for all types of pets, including dogs, cats, birds, small mammals, and exotic species. Staffers can assess whether the poison poses risk of harm to the pet, provide initial recommendations for home treatment, and, when necessary, direct you to your veterinarian for further evaluation and treatment. The help line can then provide your vet with ongoing assistance in delivering the appropriate care for your pet. There is a one-time consultation fee of $35 per incident. This fee covers not only the initial consultation, but also any follow-up consultations made with you and/or your vet.

DON'T WORRY IF YOUR PET GETS INTO ANY OF THESE

Don't be overly alarmed if your pet gets into water-based paints, plain toilet bowl water (it's icky, but it won't hurt!), silica gel, cat litter, glow jewelry, or the water in your Christmas tree container. These are considered to be nontoxic for dogs and cats, although they may cause mild gastrointestinal upset in some animals.

PETS

ALCOHOL AND ILLEGAL DRUGS

For some reason, some people think it's funny to give alcohol to a dog or cat, but this is truly dangerous. Never give your pets any alcohol or illicit drugs, and keep alcoholic beverages out of reach. Even rising bread dough can produce ethanol. Many pets have had to be treated at an emergency veterinary clinic because of the folly of their owners, and death from coma and respiratory failure is a possibility in severe cases.

SYMPTOMS OF POISONING

Signs of alcohol poisoning usually begin a half hour to an hour after ingestion, and include balance problems, vomiting, depression, disorientation, and low body temperature. High doses can lead to heart rhythm irregularities, tremors, seizures, and death.

WHAT TO DO

If you think your pet has gotten into alcohol or a drug, call the vet clinic to say you're on the way and get instructions for care during transport. If you find a chewed bottle and you aren't sure what percentage of alcohol it contained, bring it along.

ANTIFREEZE

Antifreeze (ethylene glycol) has a sweet taste that attracts pets. Even in small amounts, antifreeze is lethal to all animals, but dogs are probably most susceptible because of their tendency to taste everything. Even a tablespoon of the liquid can be toxic or fatal to a small dog, depending on the size of the animal and the concentration of the product. Cats are less likely to lap up unknown liquids, but they can walk through puddles of antifreeze on the floor, and then lick the chemical off fur or feet. Even a teaspoon can be fatal to a cat.

Although newer, pet-safe coolants are now available that contain propylene glycol or have an added bittering agent to offset the desirable taste, the traditional type of antifreeze with ethylene glycol remains the predominant coolant on the market.

SYMPTOMS OF POISONING

Antifreeze poisoning in pets progresses through three stages. First symptoms can appear within 30 minutes, and involve an appearance of drunken behavior with stumbling, staggering, vomiting, extreme thirst and frequent urination. Some animals just go to sleep, so the owners are unaware that poisoning has occurred. At the end of the first stage, the symptoms improve and the animal seems to have recovered, but during this second stage heart rate and breathing speed up. The third and final stage is unfortunately the period when problems are typically noticed; this stage progresses quickly to kidney damage, kidney failure, and coma. Signs of kidney failure include severe depression, vomiting, and diarrhea; the kidneys stop producing urine, and toxins build up in the body. Unfortunately, by the time most animals show these signs of antifreeze poisoning, it's often too late to effectively intervene.

WHAT TO DO

Antifreeze poisoning is a serious emergency that requires immediate intensive veterinary care. If you even suspect that your pet might have gotten into some antifreeze, rush him to the vet right away. If veterinary care is not immediately available, you can try to induce vomiting.

The prognosis depends on the interval between ingestion and treatment. Most dogs will recover if treated within the first eight hours; most cats will recover if treated within the first four hours.

AT THE VET'S OFFICE

If the pet has not vomited, vomiting will be induced and activated charcoal administered, followed by intravenous fluid solutions. Additional treatment depends on the stage of the disease. If your pet is not in kidney failure, the vet will give drugs to stop the metabolism of ethylene glycol into its more toxic components, or will directly remove the ethylene glycol and its metabolites from the body.

CHOCOLATE

You may have heard that chocolate can be fatal to dogs—but did you know that different chocolate products carry different risks? Chocolate contains an ingredient called theobromine (a compound similar to caffeine), but some kinds contain more theobromine than others.

Never allow your dog to eat chocolate, because all chocolate can make your dog sick, if he eats enough. Because cats are far more finicky about what they eat, they're typically much less likely to get into trouble by scarfing up a stash of chocolate. Many don't care for the taste of sweet foods at all. However, cats that do eat chocolate can become as sick as a dog would, and may require emergency care.

Unsweetened baking chocolate is the most dangerous of all chocolates, since it contains almost 10 times the amount of theobromine and caffeine as milk chocolate. Just one ounce (one square) of unsweetened baking chocolate can kill a 10-pound dog (figure about ¼ ounce for every 2.2 pounds as a fatal dose). Baker's chocolate contains 390 milligrams of theobromine per ounce. Semisweet chocolate is the next most serious threat, containing 150 milligrams of theobromine per ounce. One ounce of this type of chocolate can kill a 3-pound dog. Milk chocolate contains 44 milligrams of theobromine per ounce.

Other products that contain theobromine, caffeine, or related compounds include cocoa beans, coffee, cola, and tea, so you'll need to keep your pet away from these as well.

PREVENTION!

To prevent a poisoning incident, keep chocolate and other products containing theobromine or caffeine out of your pet's reach. Just remember: Dogs love sweets. Many are more than capable of jumping up onto a counter or table and grabbing cookies, cakes, or other chocolate temptations.

Instruct children and visitors never to feed your dog chocolate as a treat. Many people who are unaware of the danger feed their dogs candy bars or cookies without causing obvious illness—but this is only because the dose of theobromine and caffeine in small amounts of milk chocolate is relatively low, especially for larger dogs.

SYMPTOMS OF POISONING

Chocolate poisoning can cause vomiting, diarrhea, nervousness, restlessness, excitement, tremors, seizures, and even coma in dogs. Theobromine triggers the release of epinephrine (adrenaline), which makes a dog's heart race. This can progress to serious cardiac arrhythmias.

WHAT ABOUT WHITE CHOCOLATE?

Although "white chocolate" may look and taste like the real thing, it's not really chocolate at all. It's made from cocoa butter, and contains neither caffeine nor theobromine. White chocolate has no cocoa solids from the chocolate liquor, and is therefore not harmful to pets.

PETS

Theobromine and caffeine affect your pet's gastrointestinal system, central nervous system, and cardiovascular system. There is a diuretic effect as well. Symptoms include diarrhea, vomiting, increased heart rate, decreased blood pressure, restlessness, increased urination, muscle tremors, excitability, irritability, and seizures.

WHAT TO DO

Time is of the essence in these cases; seek emergency care immediately if your dog has eaten chocolate! Call your vet (or one of the animal poison control centers) immediately. Following instructions, you may be able to induce vomiting by administering hydrogen peroxide (you'll be told the correct dosage)—which greatly increases the odds of survival.

There is no specific antidote for this poisoning, so vets usually recommend inducing vomiting to get rid of the chocolate. It takes about 17.5 hours for half of the toxin in chocolate to work its way through a dog's system, so you should induce vomiting in the first one or two hours after ingestion if you don't know how much chocolate your dog ate.

HOW TO INDUCE VOMITING

In some poisoning cases, your vet or the Animal Poison Control Center will direct you to induce vomiting immediately. To make a dog vomit at home, you can force the pet to drink 3 percent household hydrogen peroxide (ask for the correct dosage, based on your pet's weight; don't guess). Keep a bottle on hand in case of emergencies, but always call a poison center or your vet before using it.

If you have activated charcoal at home, you may give your dog a dose to inhibit absorption of the toxin; the poison center will give you specific doses. In severe cases, your dog will need to be treated at the vet's office. Milk chocolate will often cause diarrhea 12 to 24 hours after ingestion. This should be treated symptomatically with fluids to prevent dehydration.

AT THE VET

Your vet may administer an anticonvulsant if neurological signs need to be controlled, along with oxygen therapy, intravenous medications, and fluids to protect the heart.

FERTILIZERS

The most serious problems resulting from fertilizer ingestion by pets are usually due to the heavy metals, such as iron, in these products. Ingestion of large amounts of fertilizer could cause severe stomach upset and possibly gastrointestinal obstruction.

WHAT TO DO

If you keep pesticides, herbicides, and fertilizers in your garage and you confine your pet in the same place, be sure to lock up these poisons. Always keep pets in mind when using these products, and keep pets off of newly treated lawns.

FLEA REPELLENT SPRAYS OR SHAMPOOS

These products may seem to be designed especially for dogs and cats, but that doesn't always make them safe. Read the warning labels carefully before using them. Some animals are particularly sensitive to the less expensive flea collars and flea products available in stores (but not the products offered by your vet).

While it may seem cost effective, never use leftover dog products on cats. Cats are much more sensitive to the toxic effects of flea and tick repellents; they are extremely sensitive to permethrin, a chemical used in more than 18 brands labeled "for dogs only." These typically contain high concentrations (45 to 65 percent) of permethrin, which are safe on dogs—but even a few drops of concentrated permethrin could be lethal to a cat. Owners most commonly expose cats to these products through inappropriate or accidental application.

SYMPTOMS OF POISONING

The signs commonly seen with permethrin toxicity in cats include general tremors and seizures. Signs can develop within hours or may take up to 48 hours to appear.

WHAT TO DO

If you've used a flea or tick product and you notice that your dog or cat seems to be acting strangely (circling, vomiting, gagging, suffering seizures), discontinue use immediately and call your vet. You may need to wash the pet to remove lingering repellent. Most pets have a good chance of recovering with prompt and aggressive veterinary treatment, including medication to control tremors and seizures, intravenous fluids, bathing, and other supportive care.

HEARTWORM

Mosquitoes can transmit the heartworm organisms (most often in dogs, and only rarely in cats), which in unvaccinated pets will grow into worms inside the body. As the worms multiply, they infest the heart and the arteries in the lungs, as well as the veins of the liver and the heart.

SYMPTOMS

The first symptoms of heartworm may not appear until a year after your dog is infected. It starts with a soft cough during exercise that gradually worsens. An infected dog will tire easily and become weak and listless to the point where he may even faint from exhaustion. He will lose weight and eventually may cough up blood. As the disease worsens, breathing becomes more difficult and the dog's quality of life will diminish drastically. Congestive heart failure and death follow.

PREVENTION!

Heartworm can be prevented with medication given once a month. A prescription medication called Revolution (selamectin) applied once a month to the skin can prevent heartworm and also kill ticks, mites, and fleas.

AT THE VET

Treatment is most likely to be successful if the disease is identified early. If the dog's heart, liver, and kidneys are still sound, the medication Immiticide will kill the worms. The treatment is given twice a day for two days, followed by several weeks of rest, so the dog's body can absorb the dead worms. It is important to keep the dog as quiet and inactive as possible, since exertion at this point can be fatal. Your vet will give you precise instructions about how much exercise your dog can have. After about a month of rest, a week of treatment will be started to kill the youngest worms.

Follow-up tests to check for the presence of heartworms should be done after one year. Surgical removal of adult heartworms may be necessary in severe cases.

HOLIDAY DECORATIONS

Although the water around the base of a Christmas tree is not deadly by itself, it may contain fertilizers that can upset a pet's stomach. In addition, stagnant tree water can be a breeding ground for bacteria.

Ribbons or tinsel can get lodged in an animal's intestines, causing obstruction. This is a very common situation for kittens, who love to play with the shiny material, but any pet might swallow tinsel.

Batteries are also often found lying around during the holidays, either to power decorations or new toys. In summer, watch out for unused fireworks, which, if ingested, can pose a danger to your pets. Many types contain potentially toxic substances such as potassium nitrate, copper, chlorates, and arsenic.

SYMPTOMS OF POISONING

A pet who drinks stagnant Christmas tree water can develop nausea, vomiting, and diarrhea. Batteries contain corrosives that can cause ulcers in the mouth, tongue, and the rest of the gastrointestinal tract if a pet swallows one.

WHAT TO DO

Take your pet to the vet if you suspect he has swallowed any type of decoration.

HOUSEPLANTS

This isn't usually too much of a problem with cats, but dogs (especially pups) like to chew, and when they're teething, they may target the family houseplants for gnawing. Some plants considered nontoxic to humans could be toxic to pets. By providing your young pet with safe, non-toxic chewable toys and snacks, you'll be helping prevent any errant—and possibly dangerous—nibbling. Many wild mushrooms are toxic (see page 101–11 for details), but it can be hard to tell which ones are which. You should assume that any mushroom your dog or cat eats is toxic, and act accordingly.

According to the ASPCA's national Animal Poison Control Center, the five most commonly reported plants that produce life-threatening problems in pets are azalea, castor bean (the source of the deadly poison ricin), lily, oleander, and sago palm. Other common plants that are toxic to pets include:

Aloe	Cyclamen	Mistletoe
Amaryllis	Dieffenbachia	Morning glory
Asparagus fern	Elephant ears	Mother-in-law
Avocado	Foxglove	tongue
Bird of paradise	Gladiola	Philodendron
Caladium	Holly	Pothos
Castor bean	Hyacinth	Tomato plant
Chinaberry tree	Iris	Tulip
Chinese evergreen	Ivy	Yew
Christmas rose	Jerusalem cherry	Yucca
Clematis	Kalanchoe	
Corn plant	Lily of the valley	
Crocus	Macadamia nut	

SYMPTOMS OF POISONING

Almost any unusual sign can be a symptom; your pet may even appear completely normal for several hours or days before showing signs of illness.

WHAT TO DO

If you catch your pet eating a plant and you don't know the exact species, take part of it to a nursery for identification.

PETS

PET-FRIENDLY PLANTS

A number of houseplants and garden plants are considered safe to have around pets. If you have household pets, plant and display on the side of safety:

Acorn squash
African violet
Bachelor's
  buttons
Bamboo
Banana tree
Begonia
Boston fern
California pitcher
  plant
Canadian
  hemlock
Canna lily
Celosia
Chaparral
Christmas palm
Cinnamon
Cinquefoil

Corn flower
Creeping Charlie
Creeping zinnia
Cucumber
Marigold
Giant aster
Gloxinia
Grape ivy
Hollyhock
Honeysuckle
Irish moss
Jasmine
Lipstick plant
Magnolia bush
Moss
Pepperomia
Poinsettia
Rubber plant

Snapdragon
Strawberry
Swedish ivy
Sweet William
Texas sage
Umbrella plant
Zinnia

LYME DISEASE

Lyme disease in dogs is transmitted just as it is in humans—via the bite of the deer tick. Ticks must be attached to an animal's skin for at least 24 hours in order to pass on the bacteria, so the sooner you see and remove ticks, the better. Lyme disease is a particular problem in dogs, although cats, cattle, and horses also can develop the disease.

PREVENTION!

A Lyme disease vaccine for dogs is 75 percent effective in preventing disease.

SYMPTOMS

Symptoms appear much differently in dogs than in humans. Dogs may develop a sudden and severe arthritis-type lameness, along with loss of appetite, fever, or vomiting. Many dogs will get severely ill very quickly. A dog can become very lethargic and refuse to move. The first stage in humans, a rash resembling a bull's eye rash, is seldom seen in dogs.

AT THE VET

Lyme disease can only be definitively diagnosed through a blood test. Luckily, prompt treatment with a month's course of the antibiotic doxycycline will eliminate the symptoms as quickly as they appeared. If the symptoms return a few weeks after the treatment is finished, retreatment may be necessary. In most cases, dogs recover completely. Untreated Lyme disease can damage the eyes, heart, kidneys, and nervous system.

MATCHES AND LIGHTER FLUID

While eating matches or lighter fluid probably won't be a problem with cats, some dogs can run into a problem if they gobble up certain types of matches that contain chlorate. Chlorate could potentially damage a dog's blood cells.

SYMPTOMS OF POISONING

Pets who eat matches can develop breathing problems or kidney

PETS

damage. Lighter fluid can irritate the skin; if ingested, it can irritate the gastrointestinal system and depress the central nervous system. Inhaled lighter fluid can lead to pneumonia and breathing problems.

WHAT TO DO

If you think your pet ate matches or drank lighter fluid, call the Animal Poison Control Center immediately for help.

MEDICATIONS

Painkillers, cold medicines, diabetes drugs, antidepressants, iron-containing vitamins, and heart drugs are common examples of human medication that could be potentially lethal to a pet even in small dosages. Most animal exposures are accidental (such as a pet chewing into a medicine bottle or eating pills left unattended or dropped on the floor), but some misguided owners try to medicate their pets without consulting a vet.

Nonsteroidal anti-inflammatory drugs (NSAIDs), a category of common painkillers that includes aspirin, ibuprofen, naproxen, and ketoprofen, are implicated in more than 4,000 pet poisonings a year.

Pseudophedrine, an ingredient found in certain cold, allergy, and sinus medications commonly used for the relief of nasal congestion in humans, can be extremely dangerous to pets. For example, as little as one tablet containing 30 milligrams of pseudoephedrine could produce symptoms in a 20-pound dog.

A dose of three 30-milligram tablets in the same dog could be lethal. From January 2003 to December 2004, the Animal Poison Control Center managed about 160 cases involving pseudoephedrine-containing products.

PREVENTION!

Sometimes people get careless about leaving medications around if there aren't any young children in the home. Never leave medications within reach of pets, and if you drop a pill, pick it up before your pet eats it. Remind guests to store their medications safely as well.

Always check with your vet before medicating pets. Many common over-the-counter medications can cause severe toxicity in both dogs and cats, even with just one tablet.

SYMPTOMS OF POISONING

Depending on the dose, NSAIDs can cause ulcers or gastrointestinal upset or perforation, bleeding disorders, kidney damage, impaired coordination, seizures, or coma. Just one 600-milligram ibuprofen tablet can be toxic to a dog of any size.

Signs of pseudophedrine poisoning are nervousness, hyperactivity and other behavioral changes, panting, rapid heart rate, and elevated blood pressure.

ONIONS AND GARLIC

Dogs or cats that eat onions or (to a lesser extent) garlic can experience serious anemia, because these foods contain thiosulphate, which is toxic to red blood cell membranes in dogs and cats. Hemolytic anemia is a condition in which the pet's red blood cells burst while circulating in its body. The red pigment from the blood cells then appears in an affected animal's urine.

All forms of onion can be a problem including dehydrated, raw, or cooked onions, onion powder, table scraps containing cooked onions, or leftovers. Even small amounts of onion may be toxic. Onion poisoning can occur after a pet eats a large amount of the food at one time, or after eating many smaller meals containing onion. A single meal of 600 to 800 grams of raw onion can be dangerous, as can multiple meals over several days containing 150 grams of onion. The pet's condition should improve once the dog no longer eats onion.

While garlic also contains the toxic ingredient thiosulphate, it is less toxic and a pet would need to eat large amounts before getting sick. Cats are believed to be a little more sensitive to onion toxicity than are dogs. Several case reports of onion toxicity suggest that onions or sizable portions of chopped onions (such as at least a cup) cause problems.

SYMPTOMS OF POISONING

A few days after eating onions or garlic, the pet will start to lose his appetite, experience stomach upset with vomiting and diarrhea, and become weak.

AT THE VET

Severe cases can require hospitalization and blood transfusions.

PESTICIDES AND HERBICIDES

Always follow label instructions when using these products, and keep your pets away from treated areas (the label will tell you for how long). In particular, the following substances are most toxic.

- Fly baits containing methomyl

- Slug and snail baits containing metaldehyde

- Systemic insecticides containing disulfoton (Di-syston) or zinc phosphide

- Strychnine in some mole or gopher bait

- Most forms of rat poison

If you've got a snail problem and you're using snail bait (metaldehyde), choose a product that doesn't look like pet food. The pellet form of this bait, in particular, is responsible for many serious pet poisonings each year. A safer bet is snail bait in the form of sawdust/powder that can be scattered in flowerbeds.

Some products designed to kill insects or mice use peanut butter as an attractant, which will interest dogs.

RAISINS AND GRAPES

Experts aren't sure why, but raisins and grapes can cause irreversible kidney failure in dogs. Cats are unlikely to eat these fruits, but if they do, they could be affected as well. Early detection and proper care can prevent serious consequences. Because experts don't know if one single large overdose is worse than an occasional nibble, the Animal Poison Control advises that pet owners not give grapes or raisins to pets in any amount.

SYMPTOMS OF POISONING
Symptoms range from vomiting to life-threatening kidney failure.

TABLE SCRAPS

It's tempting to share a morsel from your dinner plate with the pet you love, but try to resist the impulse. You should only feed animals pet food designed just for them—the fat content from table scraps can cause pancreatitis (an inflamed pancreas) in dogs. While many folks feel comfortable feeding their pets food they wouldn't eat themselves, you should never give your pet human food you think is spoiled. Animals can get sick from bad food as easily as humans.

SYMPTOMS OF POISONING
An attack of pancreatitis can be painful and cause mild vomiting,

PETS

stomach upset, abdominal pain, moodiness, and aggression. In severe attacks, it can lead to acute kidney failure and death.

AT THE VET'S OFFICE

Blood tests for pancreatic enzymes and abdominal ultrasounds, plus a medical history, can reveal the problem. Dogs with pancreatitis can't keep food or medicine down, so hospitalization with fasting, fluids, and injected painkillers and antibiotics is necessary.

XYLITOL

Contained in low-sugar or low-carbohydrate candy and gum, and some nicotine gums, the sugar alcohol known as xylitol can be toxic to pets, especially dogs. Products with the highest risk are those that list xylitol as the first or second main ingredient.

SYMPTOMS OF POISONING

Symptoms may appear within 30 minutes of eating xylitol, causing a sudden drop in blood sugar characterized by depression, lack of coordination, and seizures. Some data suggest that xylitol is also linked to liver failure in dogs.

WHAT TO DO

Xylitol poisoning is a medical emergency and requires immediate veterinary attention. Call your vet or a pet poison control center for instructions.

AT THE VET

Aggressive treatment for low blood sugar is essential.

A POISON SAFETY KIT FOR PETS

Pet owners are advised to assemble a safety kit to keep on hand for poisoning emergencies involving their animals. According to the ASPCA, this kit should contain:

✖ A fresh bottle of hydrogen peroxide, 3 percent solution (USP)

✖ Can of soft dog or cat food

✖ Turkey baster, bulb syringe, or large medical syringe

✖ Saline eye solution to flush out eye contaminants

✖ Artificial tear gel to lubricate eyes after flushing

✖ Mild grease-cutting dishwashing liquid to decontaminate skin

✖ Skunk Off! or tomato juice (for skunk spray)

✖ Rubber gloves or tough gardening gloves

✖ Forceps to remove stingers

✖ Muzzle (a frightened animal may inadvertently bite)

✖ Several soft old towels

✖ Pet carrier

11

RESOURCES

A GUIDE TO MORE INFORMATION

POISON CONTROL CENTERS IN THE UNITED STATES

The national Poison Control Center emergency number is 1-800-222-1222—it's the telephone number for every poison center in the United States. Anyone who calls this number, 24 hours a day, 7 days a week, will be connected to a poison expert. Call right away if you have a poison emergency or if you have a question about a poison or poison prevention.

The one single national poison control phone number is connected to a network of 62 poison centers around the country. When you call the number, you are connected automatically to the local poison center expert, according to the area code and exchange of the phone number you are using.

Cell phone calls also will reach a poison center. Depending on the cell phone carrier, however, you might reach the poison center in your local area or in the "home" area of the cell phone company. Either poison center can help, however.

Old numbers for local poison centers will still work, but families should post and learn the new nationwide number.

ALABAMA
Alabama Poison Center
2503 Phoenix Drive
Tuscaloosa, AL 35405
Emergency Phone: (800) 222-1222

Regional Poison Control Center
Children's Hospital
1600 7th Avenue South
Birmingham, AL 35233
Emergency Phone: (800) 222-1222

ALASKA
Oregon Poison Center
Oregon Health Sciences University
3181 S.W. Sam Jackson Park Road,
CB550
Portland, OR 97201
Emergency Phone: (800) 222-1222

ARIZONA
Arizona Poison and Drug Info Center
Arizona Health Sciences Center
Room 1156
1501 North Campbell Avenue
Tucson, AZ 85724
Emergency Phone: (800) 222-1222

Banner Poison Control Center
Good Samaritan Regional
Medical Center
1111 East McDowell
Phoenix, AZ 85006
Emergency Phone: (800) 222-1222

ARKANSAS
Arkansas Poison and Drug
Information Center
College of Pharmacy
University of Arkansas for
Medical Sciences
4301 West Markham
Mail Slot 522-2
Little Rock, AR 72205
Emergency Phone: (800) 222-1222
TDD/TTY: (800) 641-3805

CALIFORNIA
California Poison Control System—
Fresno/Madera Division
Children's Hospital Central California
9300 Valley Children's Place, MB 15
Madera, CA 93638
Emergency Phone: (800) 222-1222
TDD/TTY: (800) 972-3323

California Poison Control System—
Sacramento Division
University of California at Davis
Medical Center
2315 Stockton Boulevard
Sacramento, CA 95817
Emergency Phone: (800) 222-1222
TDD/TTY: (800) 972-3323

California Poison Control System—San
Diego Division
University of California at San Diego
Medical Center
200 West Arbor Drive
San Diego, CA 92103
Emergency Phone: (800) 222-1222
TDD/TTY: (800) 972-3323

California Poison Control System—
San Francisco Division
University of California at
San Francisco
Box 1369
San Francisco, CA 94143
Emergency Phone: (800) 222-1222
TDD/TTY: (800) 972-3323

COLORADO
Rocky Mountain Poison and
Drug Center
777 Bannock Street
Mail Code 0180
Denver, CO 80204
Emergency Phone: (800) 222-1222
TDD/TTY: (303) 739-1127

CONNECTICUT
Connecticut Poison Control Center
University of Connecticut
Health Center
263 Farmington Avenue
Farmington, CT 06030
Emergency Phone: (800) 222-1222

DELAWARE
The Poison Control Center
Children's Hospital of Philadelphia
34th Street and Civic Center Boulevard
Philadelphia, PA 19104
Emergency Phone: (800) 222-1222
TDD/TTY: (215) 590-8789

DISTRICT OF COLUMBIA
National Capital Poison Center
3201 New Mexico Avenue, N.W.
Suite 310
Washington, DC 20016
Emergency Phone: (800) 222-1222
TDD/TTY: (800) 222-1222

FLORIDA
Florida Poison Information Center—
Jacksonville
655 West Eighth Street
Jacksonville, FL 32209
Emergency Phone: (800) 222-1222
TDD/TTY: (800) 282-3171

Florida Poison Information Center—
Miami
University of Miami
Department of Pediatrics
P.O. Box 016960 (R-131)
Miami, FL 33101
Emergency Phone: (800) 222-1222

Florida Poison Information Center—
Tampa
Tampa General Hospital
P.O. Box 1289
Tampa, FL 33601
Emergency Phone: (800) 222-1222

GEORGIA
Georgia Poison Center
Hughes Spalding Children's Hospital
Grady Health System
80 Jesse Hill Jr. Drive, S.E.
P.O. Box 26066
Atlanta, GA 30335
Emergency Phone: (800) 222-1222
TDD: (404) 616-9287

HAWAII
Rocky Mountain Poison and
Drug Center
777 Bannock Street
Mail Code 0180
Denver, CO 80204
Emergency Phone: (800) 222-1222
TDD/TTY: (303) 739-1127

IDAHO
Rocky Mountain Poison and
Drug Center
777 Bannock Street
Mail Code 0180
Denver, CO 80204
Emergency Phone: (800) 222-1222
TDD/TTY: (303) 739-1127

ILLINOIS
Illinois Poison Center
222 S. Riverside Plaza, Suite 1900
Chicago, IL 60606
Emergency Phone: (800) 222-1222
TDD/TTY: (312) 906-6185

INDIANA
Indiana Poison Center
Methodist Hospital
Clarian Health Partners
I-65 at 21st Street
Indianapolis, IN 46206
Emergency Phone: (800) 222-1222
TDD/TTY: (317) 962-2336

IOWA
Iowa Statewide Poison Control Center
St. Luke's Regional Medical Center
2910 Hamilton Boulevard Lower A
Sioux City, IA 51104
Emergency Phone: (800) 222-1222

KANSAS
Mid-America Poison Control Center
University of Kansas Medical Center
3901 Rainbow Boulevard
Room B-400
Kansas City, KS 66160
Emergency Phone: (800) 222-1222
TDD/TTY: (913) 588-6639 (TDD)

KENTUCKY
Kentucky Regional Poison Center
Medical Towers South, Suite 847
234 E. Gray Street
Louisville, KY 40202
Emergency Phone: (800) 222-1222

LOUISIANA
Louisiana Drug and Poison
Information Center
University of Louisiana at Monroe
College of Pharmacy, Sugar Hall
Monroe, LA 71209
Emergency Phone: (800) 222-1222

MAINE
Northern New England Poison Center
22 Bramhall Street
Portland, ME 04102
Emergency Phone: (800) 222-1222
TDD/TTY: (877) 299-4447

MARYLAND
Maryland Poison Center
University of Maryland at Baltimore
School of Pharmacy
20 North Pine Street
Baltimore, MD 21201
Emergency Phone: (800) 222-1222
TDD/TTY: (410) 706-1858

National Capital Poison Center
3201 New Mexico Avenue, N.W.
Suite 310
Washington, DC 20016
Emergency Phone: (800) 222-1222
TDD/TTY: (800) 222-1222

MASSACHUSETTS
Regional Center for Poison Control and
Prevention Serving Massachusetts and
Rhode Island
300 Longwood Avenue
Boston, MA 02115
Emergency Phone: (800) 222-1222
TDD/TTY: (888) 244-5313

MICHIGAN
Children's Hospital of Michigan
Regional Poison Control Center
4160 John R. Harper Professional
Office Building, Suite 616
Detroit, MI 48201
Emergency Phone: (800) 222-1222
TDD/TTY: (800) 356-3232

DeVos Children's Hospital Regional
Poison Center
1300 Michigan, N.E., Suite 203
Grand Rapids, MI 49503
Emergency Phone: (800) 222-1222
TDD/TTY: (800) 222-1222

MINNESOTA
Hennepin Regional Poison Center
Hennepin County Medical Center
701 Park Avenue
Minneapolis, MN 55415
Emergency Phone: (800) 222-1222
TDD/TTY: (612) 904-4691

MISSISSIPPI
Mississippi Regional Poison
Control Center
University of Mississippi
Medical Center
2500 N. State Street
Jackson, MS 39216
Emergency Phone: (800) 222-1222

MISSOURI
Missouri Regional Poison Center
7980 Clayton Road, Suite 200
St. Louis, MO 63117
Emergency Phone: (800) 222-1222
TDD/TTY: (314) 612-5705

MONTANA
Rocky Mountain Poison and Drug
Center
777 Bannock Street
Mail Code 0180
Denver, CO 80204
Emergency Phone: (800) 222-1222
TDD/TTY: (303) 739-1127

NEBRASKA
Nebraska Regional Poison Center
8200 Dodge Street
Omaha, NE 68114
Emergency Phone: (800) 222-1222

NEVADA

Oregon Poison Center

Oregon Health Sciences University
3181 S.W. Sam Jackson Park Road,
CB550
Portland, OR 97201
Emergency Phone: (800) 222-1222

Rocky Mountain Poison and Drug Center

777 Bannock Street
Mail Code 0180
Denver, CO 80204
Emergency Phone: (800) 222-1222
TDD/TTY: (303) 739-1127

NEW HAMPSHIRE

New Hampshire Poison Information
Center

Dartmouth-Hitchcock Medical Center
One Medical Center Drive
Lebanon, NH 03756
Emergency Phone: (800) 222-1222

NEW JERSEY

New Jersey Poison Information and
Education System

University of Medicine and Dentistry
of New Jersey
65 Bergen Street
Newark, NJ 07107
Emergency Phone: (800) 222-1222
TDD/TTY: (973) 926-8008

NEW MEXICO

New Mexico Poison and Drug Info Center

Health Science Center Library,
Room 130
University of New Mexico
Albuquerque, NM 87131
Emergency Phone: (800) 222-1222

NEW YORK

Central New York Poison Center

750 E. Adams Street
Syracuse, NY 13210
Emergency Phone: (800) 222-1222

Finger Lakes Regional Poison and Drug
Information Center

University of Rochester
Medical Center
601 Elmwood Avenue, Box 321
Rochester, NY 14642
Emergency Phone: (800) 222-1222
TDD/TTY: (585) 273-3854

Long Island Regional Poison and Drug
Information Center

Winthrop University Hospital
259 First Street
Mineola, NY 11501
Emergency Phone: (800) 222-1222
TDD/TTY: (516) 924-8811 (Suffolk);
(516) 747-3323 (Nassau)

New York City Poison Control Center

New York City Bureau of Labs
455 First Avenue, Room 123, Box 81
New York, NY 10016
Emergency Phone: (800) 222-1222
TDD/TTY: (212) 689-9014

Western New York Poison Center
Children's Hospital of Buffalo
219 Bryant Street
Buffalo, NY 14222
Emergency Phone: (800) 222-1222

NORTH CAROLINA

Carolinas Poison Center
Carolinas Medical Center
5000 Airport Center Parkway, Suite B
Charlotte, NC 28208
Emergency Phone: (800) 222-1222

NORTH DAKOTA

Hennepin Regional Poison Center
Hennepin County Medical Center
701 Park Avenue
Minneapolis, MN 55415
Emergency Phone: (800) 222-1222
TDD/TTY: (612) 904-4691

OHIO

Central Ohio Poison Center
700 Children's Drive, Room L032
Columbus, OH 43205
Emergency Phone: (800) 222-1222
TDD/TTY: (614) 228-2272

Cincinnati Drug and Poison
Information Center
3333 Burnet Avenue
Vernon Place, 3rd Floor
Cincinnati, OH 45229
Emergency Phone: (800) 222-1222
TDD/TTY: (800) 253-7955

Greater Cleveland Poison Control Center
11100 Euclid Avenue
Cleveland, OH 44106
Emergency Phone: (800) 222-1222

OKLAHOMA

Oklahoma Poison Control Center
Children's Hospital at Oklahoma
University Medical Center
940 N.E. 13th Street, Room 3510
Oklahoma City, OK 73104
Emergency Phone: (800) 222-1222
TDD/TTY: (405) 271-1122

OREGON

Oregon Poison Center
Oregon Health Sciences University
3181 S.W. Sam Jackson Park Road,
CB550
Portland, OR 97201
Emergency Phone: (800) 222-1222

PENNSYLVANIA

Pittsburgh Poison Center
Children's Hospital of Pittsburgh
3705 Fifth Avenue
Pittsburgh, PA 15213
Emergency Phone: (800) 222-1222

The Poison Control Center
Children's Hospital of Philadelphia
34th and Civic Center Boulevard
Philadelphia, PA 19104
Emergency Phone: (800) 222-1222
TDD/TTY: (215) 590-8789

PUERTO RICO
Puerto Rico Poison Center
Calle San Jorge #252
Santurce, PR 00912
Emergency Phone: (800) 222-1222

RHODE ISLAND
Regional Center for Poison Control and
Prevention Serving Massachusetts and
Rhode Island
300 Longwood Avenue
Boston, MA 02115
Emergency Phone: (800) 222-1222
TDD/TTY: (888) 244-5313

SOUTH CAROLINA
Palmetto Poison Center
College of Pharmacy
University of South Carolina
Columbia, SC 29208
Emergency Phone: (800) 222-1222

SOUTH DAKOTA
Hennepin Regional Poison Center
Hennepin County Medical Center
701 Park Avenue
Minneapolis, MN 55415
Emergency Phone: (800) 222-1222
TDD/TTY: (612) 904-4691

TENNESSEE
Middle Tennessee Poison Center
501 Oxford House
1161 21st Avenue S.
Nashville, TN 37232
Emergency Phone: (800) 222-1222
TDD/TTY: (615) 936-2047

TEXAS
Central Texas Poison Center
Scott and White Memorial Hospital
2401 South 31st Street
Temple, TX 76508
Emergency Phone: (800) 222-1222

North Texas Poison Center
Parkland Memorial Hospital
5201 Harry Hines Boulevard
Dallas, TX 75235
Emergency Phone: (800) 222-1222

Southeast Texas Poison Center
The University of Texas
Medical Branch
3.112 Trauma Building
Galveston, TX 77555-1175
Emergency Phone: (800) 222-1222

South Texas Poison Center
The University of Texas Health
Science Center—San Antonio
Department of Surgery
Mail Code 7849
7703 Floyd Curl Drive
San Antonio, TX 78229
Emergency Phone: (800) 222-1222

Texas Panhandle Poison Center
1501 South Coulter
Amarillo, TX 79106
Emergency Phone: (800) 222-1222

West Texas Regional Poison Center
Thomason Hospital
4815 Alameda Avenue
El Paso, TX 79905
Emergency Phone: (800) 222-1222

UTAH
Utah Poison Control Center
585 Komas Drive, Suite 200
Salt Lake City, UT 84108
Emergency Phone: (800) 222-1222

VERMONT
Northern New England Poison Center
22 Bramhall Street
Portland, ME 04102
Emergency Phone: (800) 222-1222
TDD/TTY: (207) 871-2879

VIRGINIA
Blue Ridge Poison Center
Jefferson Park Place
1222 Jefferson Park Avenue
Charlottesville, VA 22903
Emergency Phone: (800) 222-1222

National Capital Poison Center
3201 New Mexico Avenue, N.W.
Suite 310
Washington, DC 20016
Emergency Phone: (800) 222-1222
TDD/TTY: (800) 222-1222

Virginia Poison Center
Medical College of Virginia Hospitals
Virginia Commonwealth University
Health System
P.O. Box 980522
Richmond, VA 23298
Emergency Phone: (800) 222-1222

WASHINGTON
Washington Poison Center
155 N.E. 100th Street, Suite 400
Seattle, WA 98125
Emergency Phone: (800) 222-1222
TDD/TTY: (206) 517-2394;
(800) 572-0638 (Washington only)

WEST VIRGINIA
West Virginia Poison Center
3110 MacCorkle Avenue, S.E.
Charleston, WV 25304
Emergency Phone: (800) 222-1222
TDD/TTY: (304) 388-9698

WISCONSIN
Children's Hospital of Wisconsin
Poison Center
P.O. Box 1997, Mail Station 677A
Milwaukee, WI 53201
Emergency Phone: (800) 222-1222
TDD/TTY: (414) 266-2542

WYOMING
Nebraska Regional Poison Center
8200 Dodge Street
Omaha, NE 68114
Emergency Phone: (800) 222-1222

ORGANIZATIONS

American Association of
Poison Control Centers
3201 New Mexico Avenue, Suite 330
Washington, DC 20016
(202) 362-7217
www.aapcc.org

Consumer Product Safety Commission
4330 East-West Highway
Bethesda, MD 20814
(800) 638-2772
www.cpsc.gov

National Environmental Health
Association (NEHA)
National Radon Proficiency Program
P.O. Box 2109
Fletcher, NC 28732
(800) 269-4174 or (828) 890-4117
E-mail: angel@neha-nrpp.org
www.neha-nrpp.org

National Institute of Environmental
Health Sciences
111 Alexander Drive
Research Triangle Park, NC 27709
(919) 541-3345
www.niehs.nih.gov

National Lead Information Center
Clearinghouse
(800) 424-5323 (424-LEAD)

National Radon Safety Board (NRSB)
14 Hayes Street
Elmsford, NY 10523
(866) 329-3474
E-mail: info@nrsb.org
www.nrsb.org

POISON EDUCATION AND INFORMATION MATERIALS

HOME SAFETY
Home Safety Checklist
American Academy of Pediatrics
37925 Eagle Way
Chicago, IL 60678
(888) 227-1770
Fax: (847) 228-1281
www.aap.org/bookstore
This "full-house" checklist enables parents to identify potential safety risks inside and outdoors. Sold in pads of 100 for $19.95 (members, $14.95) plus $5.95 for shipping and handling.

LEAD POISONING
Protect Your Family from Lead in Your Home
U.S. Consumer Product Safety Commission
Washington, DC 20207
E-mail: publications@cpsc.gov
www.cpsc.gov/cpscpub/pubs/426.html
Request a free booklet about the dangers of lead-based paint, testing the paint in your home for lead, and ways to reduce your exposure, via the e-mail address above.

Lead Screening for Children
American Academy of Pediatrics
37925 Eagle Way
Chicago, IL 60678
(888) 227-1770
Fax: (847) 228-1281
www.aap.org/bookstore
This educational brochure gives parents vital guidelines on how to identify and eliminate the dangerous sources of lead poisoning in the home. It also provides clear information on how to recognize the symptoms of lead poisoning in children. Sold in packs of 100 for $35.95 (members, $30) plus $7.95 for shipping and handling.

MEDICATIONS
A Guide to Children's Medications
American Academy of Pediatrics
37925 Eagle Way
Chicago, IL 60678
(888) 227-1770
Fax: (847) 228-1281
www.aap.org/bookstore
This brochure helps eliminate confusion about the differences between common prescription and over-the-counter medications. Includes information on taking medications correctly and safely. Sold in packs of 100 for $35 (members, $30) plus $7.95 for shipping and handling.

National Safe Kids Campaign Resources
National Safe Kids Campaign
1301 Pennsylvania Avenue, N.W.
Suite 1000
Washington, DC 20004
(202) 662-0600
E-mail: info@safekids.org
www.safekids.org
Offers a poison injury fact sheet, a brochure for adults, and a children's booklet, "Filbert Prevents a Poison."

Mr. Yuk Stickers and Related Materials
Poison Education Materials

Pittsburgh Poison Center
3705 Fifth Avenue
Pittsburgh, PA 15213
(412) 692-5315
Fax: (412) 390-3311
Each sheet of generic Mr. Yuk stickers contains 10 individual stickers and has the words "Poison Help" and 1-800-222-1222. A description of each item and information on how to order materials can be found at www.chp.edu/mryuk/05d_yukkygame.php.

NONTOXIC ART MATERIALS
What You Need to Know about the Safety of Art and Craft Materials
Art and Creative Materials Institute
P.O. Box 479
Hanson, MA 02341
(781) 293-4100
Fax: (781) 294-0808
www.acminet.org
Contact the organization to obtain a free 12-page booklet that answers commonly asked questions about the safe use of art materials.

PESTICIDES/CHEMICALS
Pesticides and Child Safety
National Service Center for Environmental Publications
P.O. Box 42419
Cincinnati, OH 45242
(800) 490-9198
www.epa.gov/ncepihom
Free copies of tips on safeguarding children from accidental pesticide poisoning or exposure and important contact phone numbers if an accident occurs. The National Service Center for Environmental Publications maintains and distributes EPA publications in paper, CD-ROM, and other multi-media formats. The current publication inventory includes more than 7,000 titles.

To order EPA publications, you will need the publication number: EPA #735-F-93-050. The publication is also available in Spanish.

Ten Tips to Protect Children from Pesticide and Lead Poisoning around the Home
National Service Center for Environmental Publications
P.O. Box 42419
Cincinnati, OH 45242
(800) 490-9198
www.epa.gov/ncepihom
Free copies. The National Service Center for Environmental Publications maintains and distributes EPA publications in paper, CD-ROM, and other multi-media formats. The current publication inventory includes more than 7,000 titles. To order EPA publications, you will need the publication number: EPA #735-F-93-001.

Read the Label First! Protect Your Kids
National Service Center for Environmental Publications
P.O. Box 42419
Cincinnati, OH 45242
(800) 490-9198
www.epa.gov/ncepihom
Free brochure about protecting children from exposure to household cleaners and pesticides. The National Service Center for Environmental Publications maintains and distributes EPA publications in paper, CD-ROM, and other multi-media formats. The current publication inventory includes more than 7,000 titles. To order EPA publications, you will need the publication number: #740-F-00-001.

PET POISONING
Animal Poison Control Center Magnet
www.aspca.org/site/PageServer?

pagename=pro_apcc_magnet
You can get a free animal poison control center magnet that displays the center's phone number by filling out the form online at the address above.

PLANTS
Plants That Poison

Bronson Hospital Poison Prevention
601 John Street, Box 56
Kalamazoo, MI 49007
Obtain a free illustrated chart of common poisonous plants—indicating size, toxic parts, and symptoms of poisoning—with information on preventing plant poisoning and emergency measures by sending a self-addressed, stamped business envelope to the address above.

POISON PREVENTION
Poison Prevention Community Action Kit

National Safety Council
1025 Connecticut Avenue, N.W.
Suite 1200
Washington, DC 20036
This free 3-ring binder includes fact sheets, outreach materials and opportunities, PowerPoint presentations, Web pages, children's activities, and information on presenting your activities to the media. The information is available both in hard copy and on a CD-ROM designed so you can customize the information by placing your own contact information on it.

"Locked Up Poisons"
Poison Prevention Week Council
P.O. Box 1543
Washington, DC 20013
E-mail: kdulic@cpsc.gov
www.cpsc.gov/cpscpub/pubs/382.html
This document is free. You may download it or obtain hard copies from the address above. Also available in Spanish.

National Poison Prevention Week Packet
Poison Prevention Week Council
P.O. Box 1543
Washington, DC 20013
E-mail: kdulic@cpsc.gov
A folder containing a list of available materials, a fact sheet, and other promotional materials for the annual National Poison Prevention Week observance (the third week of March).

SAFETY ISSUES
TIPP Safety Slips

American Academy of Pediatrics
37925 Eagle Way
Chicago, IL 60678
(888) 227-1770
Fax: (847) 228-1281
www.aap.org/bookstore
Topic-specific sheets on safety that focus on frequent causes of childhood injuries and simple ways to prevent them. $5^1/_2$ x $8^1/_2$" sheets. Each of the 14 child safety slips provides guidelines for the prevention of injury hazards. Included: Babysitting Reminders; Safety Tips for Home Playground Equipment; Protect Your Child...Prevent Poisoning; When Your Child Needs Emergency Medical Services. Components sold in packs of 100 for $24.95 (members, $19.95) plus $5.95 for shipping and handling.

MEDIA

FILMS, SLIDES, TALKS, AND
MEDIA AIDS

The Travels of Timothy Trent

National Technical Information Service
National Audiovisual Center
5285 Port Royal Road
Springfield, VA 22161
(800) 553-6847
www.ntis.gov/search/product.asp?
ABBR=AVA03690VNB1

A short film showing how poison preventive packaging provides an additional safety margin against accidental poisoning in children. Demonstrates the point through Timothy Trent, a young boy who can't resist putting everything he can reach in his mouth. Price is $50.

Poison Proof Your Home

Hyper.Active Media and Content Inc.
1240 Bay Street, Suite 500
Toronto, Ontario M5R 2A7
(416) 324-1771

This 30-minute interactive video shows how to prevent child poisonings. Presents a room-by-room and step-by-step outline of what hazardous substances can exist in a typical household and how to store and safely destroy them. Price is $20, including shipping and handling.

POSTERS

3-in-1 First Aid, Choking, CPR Chart

American Academy of Pediatrics
37925 Eagle Way
Chicago, IL 60678
(888) 227-1770
Fax: (847) 228-1281
www.aap.org/bookstore

This quick guide helps you respond rapidly and effectively in emergencies. Large wall chart includes first aid guidance on one side with choking/CPR guidance on the other. Topics include burns, scalds, fractures, sprains, head injuries, poisons, skin wounds, stings and bites, and infant/child CPR. Single copy price $2.95; pack of 100 is $55 (members, $49) plus $9.95 for shipping and handling.

National Poison Prevention Week

Poison Prevention Week Council
P.O. Box 1543
Washington, DC 20013
E-mail: kdulic@cpsc.gov

For the latest tips, posters, and other information, contact the Poison Prevention Week Council at the above address. The publications are updated yearly. All items are also available in Spanish.

INDEX

Note: *Italic* page numbers refer to illustrations.

acetaminophen, 37–39, 46
activated charcoal, 26–27
alcohol, 157–58, 268
allergies
    to bee stings, 126, 130, 131
    to mushrooms, 103
    to poison ivy, 97
aluminum phosphide, 176–77
anisakiasis, 212, 214
antianxiety drugs, 39–40
anticonvulsant drugs, 40–41
antidepressants, 41–42
antifreeze, 30, 158–59, 170–71, 265, 268–70
anti-inflammatory drugs (NSAIDS), 43, 47, 280
antique toys, 257
art supplies, 17, 18, 251–53, 254, 255, 257
ASPCA Animal Poison Control Center, 266
aspirin, 44–45
asthma, 29, 49, 135, 233
at-home antidotes, 25, 26, 27
automatic dishwasher soap, 159–60
autumn crocus, 71–72
azalea/rhododendron, 66–67, *66*, 277

bacillus cereus, 212, 215
bathroom, 29–30
batteries, 30, 162, 276
bees and wasps, 126–32, *126*
belladonna, 92–93
benzene, 168–70
beta blockers, 48–49
birth control pills, 45
black widow spider, 148–49, *148*
bleach, 28, 161–62
blood pressure medication, 45–46

blood transfusions, 146
botulism, 211, 212, 215–18
brown recluse spider, 150–51, *150*
buck moth caterpillar, 135–36
bufo toad, 122–23, *122*
bullets, lead in, 258–59
button batteries, 30, 162

caladium, 89
calcium channel blockers, 49
campylobacteriosis, 212, 218–20, 220
canebrake rattler, 118, *118*
carbamates, 175
carbon monoxide, 162–66
caterpillars, *133*
    buck moth caterpillar, 135–36
    first aid for stings, 134–35
    hagmoth caterpillar, 136
    hickory tussock caterpillar, 136–37
    io moth caterpillar, 137
    prevention of stings, 133–34
    puss caterpillar, 138
    saddleback caterpillar, 138–39
    silverspotted tiger moth caterpillar, 139
    stinging rose caterpillar, 139–40
catfish, 186, *186*
caustics, 166–68
ceramics, lead in, 255
chaparral, 59
chemicals
    alcohol, 157–58
    antifreeze, 30, 158–59, 170–71, 265, 268–70
    automatic dishwasher soap, 159–60
    batteries, 30, 162, 276
    bleach, 28, 161–62
    carbon monoxide, 162–66
    caustics, 166–68
    children and, 155–56, 250
    hydrocarbons, 168–70
    methanol, 170–71
    mixing of, 28

mouthwash, 171–72
paint (oil-based), 172–73
pesticides, 31, 156, 173–78, 265,
  273, 282
playground equipment, 178–80
storage of, 30, 156, 158–59
swimming pool cleaners, 182–83
childproof safety latches, 31
children. *See also* infants; nursery/
  playroom safety
accidental poisonings and, 17–19
chemicals and, 155–56, 250
child-safe plants, 65
lead poisoning and, 253–54
child-resistant caps, 29, 34, 51
child-resistant packaging, 173
chimneys, 165
chinaberry tree, 67–68, *67*, 277
chocolate, and pets, 270–73
Christmas rose, 68–69, *68*
cigarette butts, 30
ciguatera, 212, 220–22
cleaning products, 28–29, 166–68,
  182–83, 251
clematis, 70, *70*, 277
codeine, 55
cold medications, 46–47
comfrey, 59
Consumer Product Safety Commission,
  26, 178–79, 257
contaminated soil, 254, 261
copperheads, 120, *120*
coprine class of mushrooms, 103–4,
  103
coral snakes, 114–15, 120–21, *121*
costume/toy jewelry, lead in, 256
cottonmouth, 193–95, *193*
CPR, 19, 25, 26
crocus, autumn, 71–72, *71*, 277
cryptosporidiosis, 212, 222–24
curtain weights, lead in, 256
cyclopeptide class of mushrooms,
  104–5, 104

cyclosporiasis, 212, 224–25

daffodil, 90–91
death camas, 72–73, *72*
dieffenbachia, 73–74
digoxin, 49
diquat, 177–78
drain cleaners, 166–68
dumbcane, 73–74, *73*
duplicating fluid, 170–71

eastern coral snake, 121, *121*
eastern diamondback rattlesnake, 117,
  117
E. coli, 211, 212, 225–28
egg safety, 210, 237
Environmental Protection Agency, 156,
  173, 180, 255
ephedra, 59
eucalyptus oil, 59
eye exposure
  automatic dishwasher soap and, 160
  bleach and, 162
  bufo toad and, 123
  caustics and, 168
  first aid for, 25
  swimming pool cleaners and, 183

fertilizers, and pets, 273
fireplaces, 166
first aid
  knowledge of, 19
  for poisoning, 25–28
fish. *See also* meat; poultry; water
    creatures
  anisakiasis and, 214
  ciguatera and, 220–22
  food poisoning prevention and,
    199–201
  hepatitis A and, 231, 232
  listeriosis and, 234
  shellfish poisoning, 213, 238–41
  shopping for, 199–201

storage times for, 200
vibrio and, 246
flea repellant, 273–74
folk remedies, 61
Food and Drug Administration (FDA),
    57–58, 257
food poisoning. *See also specific types*
    chart of types, 212–13
    food-borne illness, 210–11
    food preparation and, 204–6,
        208–10
    incidence of, 197–98
    prevention of, 198–204
    reporting of, 207
    treatment of, 210–11
food preparation, 204–6, 208–10, 220
food storage, 28, 202–4, 206, 208
formaldehyde, 168–70
foxglove, 74–76, *74*, 277
furniture polish, 168–70

garages/sheds, 30–31, 170
garlic, and pets, 281–82
gasoline, 168–70
gas or oil furnaces, 165
gastrointestinal irritant class of
    mushrooms, 105–6, *105*
germander, 60
giardiasis, 212, 228–31
grapes, and pets, 283
Guillain-Barré syndrome, 219

hagmoth caterpillar, 136
hallucinogenic class of mushrooms,
    106–7, *106*
handbags, 30, 34
hand washing
    and bufo toad, 123
    campylobacteriosis and, 220
    cryptosporidiosis and, 223
    food preparation and, 204
    giardiasis and, 229
    lead poisoning and, 260

listeriosis and, 234
salmonellosis and, 237
shigellosis and, 241
heart medications, 48–51
heartworm, 274–75
heating-unit venting systems, 165
heavy metals. *See also* lead
    herbal products and, 57, 61
    oil-based paint and, 172
    pets and, 273
hemlock, poison, 76–77, *76*
hepatitis A, 213, 231–33
herbal products, 56–61
herbicides, 30, 273
hickory tiger caterpillar, 136–3
hobbies, lead in, 254
holiday decorations, 276
holly, 77–78, *77*, 277
home canning, 216
honey, 218
houseplants, 30, 63, 65, 94–95,
    276–78
hyacinth, 78–79, *78*, 277
hydrocarbons, 168–70
hydrocodone, 5

ibuprofen, 43
infants. *See also* nursery/playroom
        safety
    botulism and, 218
    chemicals and, 250, 251
    keeping babies clean, 263
    salmonellosis and, 238
    toxoplasmosis and, 244
inhalation of toxic fumes/gases
    art supplies and, 253
    bleach and, 161
    carbon monoxide and, 163
    first aid for, 25
    hydrocarbons and, 169
    methanol and, 170–71
    painting and, 256
    rat poison and, 176

swimming pool cleaners and, 182
insecticides, 30
insects
    bees and wasps, 126–32
    caterpillars, 133–40
    mosquitoes, 144–47
    prevention of stinging, 125, 127–28
    scorpions, 151–53
    spiders, 148–51
    ticks, 140–44
insect sting allergy kit, 131
io moth caterpillar, 137
ipecac, syrup of, 27–28
iron, in drugs and supplements, 29,
    50–52
isoniazid, 52–53
ivy, 79–80, *79*, 27

jack-in-the-pulpit, 80–81, *80*
jellyfish, 187–89, *187*
Jerusalem cherry, 81–82, *81*, 277
jessamine, 82, *82*
jimsonweed, 83–84, *83*
jonquil, 90–91

kava, 60
kerosene, 168–70
killer bees, 132
kitchen, 28–29
kohl, lead in, 258

lamp oil, 168–70
laundry, 28–29
leaded crystal, 258
lead poisoning
    art supplies and, 251, 254, 255,
        257
    causes of, 253–54
    herbal products and, 57, 61
    infants and, 250
    information on, 262
    prevention of, 260–61
    screening for, 261

sources of, 254–59
    symptoms of, 259
    treatment of, 260
lead solder, 255
lighter fluid, 168–70, 279–80
lily of the valley, 84–85, *84*, 277
lindane, 174
lion's mane, 187
listeriosis, 213, 233–35
living room/family room, 30
Lyme disease, 140, 141, 142–43, 144,
    278–79
Lyme disease vaccine for dogs, 141,
    279

mad cow disease, 235–36
ma-huang, 59
matches, 279–80
meat. *See also* fish; poultry
    cooking temperature, 206
    E. coli poisoning and, 211, 225–26
    freezer storage tips, 203–4
    listeriosis and, 233
    mad cow disease and, 235–36
    salmonellosis and, 237
    shopping for, 201–2
    thawing, 206
    toxoplasmosis and, 243
    trichinellosis and, 244–45
media resources, 301
medications
    accidental overdose and, 33–36
    acetaminophen, 37–39, 46
    antianxiety drugs, 39–40
    anticonvulsant drugs, 40–41
    antidepressants, 41–42
    anti-inflammatory drugs (NSAIDS),
        43, 47, 280
    aspirin, 44–45
    birth control pills, 45
    blood pressure medication, 45–46
    cold medications, 46–47
    giving medicine safely, 35–36

heart medications, 48–51
herbal products, 56–61
iron in, 50–52
isoniazid, 52–53
metformin, 53
methylphenidate, 54
opioids (narcotics), 55
pets and, 280–81
storage of, 29, 34–35
thyroid medication, 56
mercury, 57
metformin, 53
methadone, 55
methanol, 170–71
methylphenidate, 54
Mexican candies, lead in, 258
milk
    campylobacteriosis and, 218, 219,
        220
    E. coli and, 226
    listeriosis and, 233, 234
mistletoe, 85–86, 85, 277
Mojave rattler, 119, *119*
monkshood, 86–88, *86*
monomethylhydrazine class of
        mushrooms, 107–8, *107*
morning glory, 88–89, *88*, 277
morphine, 55
mosquitoes, 144–47, 274–75
mother-in-law plant, 89, *89*
motor oil, 168–70
mouthwash, 171–72
muscarine class of mushrooms, 108–9,
        108
muscimol/ibotenic acid class of
        mushrooms, 109–10, *109*
mushrooms, poisonous
    coprine class, 103–4
    cyclopeptide class, 104–5
    gastrointestinal irritant class, 105–6
    hallucinogenic class, 106–7
    monomethylhydrazine class, 107–8
    muscarine class, 108–9

muscimol/ibotenic acid class,
    109–10
orelline class, 110–11
symptoms of poisoning, 101–2

narcissus, 90–91, *90*
narcotics (opioids), 55
nightshade, black, 91–92, *91*
nightshade, deadly, 92–93, *92*
NSAIDS (anti-inflammatory drugs), 43,
    47, 280
nursery/playroom safety
    and art supplies, 251–53, 254, 255,
        257
    lead poisoning and, 253–62
    nontoxic substances in, 250
    talcum powder and, 262–63

oil of wintergreen, 60
oleander, white and yellow, 93–94, *93*,
    277
onions, and pets, 281–82
opioids (narcotics), 55
orelline class of mushrooms, 110–11,
    110
organochlorines, 174–75
organophosphates, 175
oven cleaners, 166–68
oxycodone, 55

Pacific rattler, 119, *119*
paint (lead-based), 253–54, 257, 260
paint (oil-based), 172–73
paint removers, 170–71
paint thinners, 168–70
paraquat, 177–78
pennyroyal, 60
perfumes, 170–71
pesticides
    organochlorines, 174–75
    organophosphates, 175
    pets and, 273, 282
    poison prevention and, 31, 156

pyrethrins, 176
rat poisons, 176–77, 265
sources of exposure, 173
weed killer, 177–78
Pet Poison HELPLINE, 266–67
pets
alcohol and, 268
antifreeze and, 158, 265, 268–70
carbon monoxide and, 166
chocolate and, 270–73
fertilizers and, 273
flea repellant and, 273–74
heartworm and, 274–75
holiday decorations and, 276
houseplants and, 276–78
Lyme disease and, 141, 278–79
matches and lighter fluid and,
279–80
medications and, 280–81
nontoxic substances and, 267
onions and garlic and, 281–82
pesticides and, 273, 282
Pet Poison HELPLINE, 266–67
poison safety kit for, 285
raisins and grapes and, 283
table scraps and, 283–84
toxoplasmosis and, 243
xylitol and, 284
philodendron, 94–95, 277
plant poisoning
azalea/rhododendron, 66–67, 277
causes of, 64
child-safe plants, 65
chinaberry tree, 67–68, 277
Christmas rose, 68–69
clematis, 70, 277
crocus, autumn, 71–72, 277
death camas, 72–73
dumbcane, 73–74
foxglove, 74–76, 277
hemlock, poison, 76–77
holly, 77–78, 277
houseplants and, 30, 63, 65,

94–95, 276–78
hyacinth, 78–79, 277
ivy, 79–80, 277
jack-in-the-pulpit, 80–81
Jerusalem cherry, 81–82, 277
jessamine, 82
jimsonweed, 83–84
lily of the valley, 84–85, 277
mistletoe, 85–86, 277
monkshood, 86–88
morning glory, 88–89, 277
mother-in-law plant, 89
mushrooms, 101–11
narcissus, 90–91
nightshade, black, 91–92
nightshade, deadly, 92–93
oleander, white and yellow, 93–94,
277
philodendron, 94–95, 277
poison ivy, oak, and sumac, 95–98
tomato plant, 99–100, 277
playground equipment, 178–80
poinsettia, 65
Poison Control Centers, 19, 23–24, 36,
288–96
poison education, 298–300
poisoning. *See also* food poisoning; lead
poisoning; plant poisoning
basics of, 21–31
first aid for, 25–28
prevention of, 28–31
response to, 23–24
signs of, 22
poison ivy, 95–98, *95*
poison oak, 95–98, *95*
poison organizations, 297
poison sumac, 95–98, *95*
pool cue chalk, lead in, 257
Portuguese man-of-war, 187
poultry. *See also* fish; meat
campylobacteriosis and, 218, 219,
220
cooking temperature, 206

freezer storage tips, 203–4
salmonellosis and, 237
shopping for, 201–2
thawing, 206
pressure-treated wood, 178–80
projectiles, lead in, 258–59
protective clothing, 31
puss caterpillar, 138
pyrethrins and synthetic pyrethroids, 176

radon, 180–82
raisins, and pets, 283
rat poisons, 176–77, 265
rattlesnakes
canebrake rattler, 118
eastern diamondback, 117
Mojave rattler, 119
Pacific rattler, 119
sidewinder, 119–20
symptoms of poisoning, 117
timber rattler, 118
types of, 116
western diamondback, 117–18
refrigeration, 203–4
Reye's syndrome, 37, 44
rhododendron, 66–67, 277
rhubarb, 98–99, *98*
Ritalin, 54

salmonellosis, 213, 237–38
sassafras, 60
scorpions, 151–53, *151*
sea anemones, 190–91, *190*
seafood. *See* fish
sea nettles, 187
sea urchins, 191–92, *191*
"sell by" date, 199, 202
shellac, 170–71
shellfish poisoning, 213, 238–41
shigellosis, 213, 241–42
shopping
for fish, 199–201

food poisoning prevention and, 198–99
for meat and poultry, 201–2
sidewinder, 119–20, *119*
silverspotted tiger moth caterpillar, 139
skin exposure
art supplies and, 253
automatic dishwasher soap and, 160
bleach and, 162
bufo toad and, 123
catfish stings and, 186
caustics and, 168
first aid for, 25
jellyfish stings and, 187–88
methanol and, 170
swimming pool cleaners and, 182, 183
snail bait, and pets, 265, 282–83
snakes
copperheads, 120
coral snakes, 114–15, 120–21
first aid for snakebite, 115–16
hospital treatment for snakebite, 116
pit vipers, 114
rattlesnakes, 116–20
symptoms of poisoning from snakebite, 117, 120, 121
treating bites as medical emergency, 113, 115
water moccasins, 193–95
solvents, 170–71
spiders
black widow spider, 148–49
brown recluse spider, 150–51
staphylococcal food poisoning, 213, 242–43
stinging rose caterpillar, 139–40
stingrays, 192–93, *192*
storage
of chemicals, 30, 156, 158–59
food storage, 28, 202–4, 206, 208
of medications, 29, 34–35
stove pilot lights, 166